ABC OF ORAL HEALTH

Edited by

CRISPIAN SCULLY CBE

Dean, Director of Studies and Research,
Eastman Dental Institute for Oral Health Care Sciences,
University College London, University of London, UK

BMJ
Books

BMJ Books is an imprint of the BMJ Publishing Group

First published in 2001
by BMJ Books, BMA House, Tavistock Square,
London WC1H 9JR

www.bmjbooks.com

British Library Cataloguing in Publication Data
A catalogue record for this book is available from the British Library

ISBN 0-7279-1551-7

Cover design by Marritt Associates, Harrow, Middlesex
Composition by Scribe Design, Gillingham, Kent
Printed and bound in Spain by GraphyCems, Navarra

Contents

Contributors

Raman Bedi
Professor of Transcultural Oral Health

John Coventry
Senior Lecturer in Periodontology

Susan Cunningham
Lecturer

Roger Davies
Consultant in Special Needs Dentistry

Brigitte Griffiths
Consultant

Gareth Griffiths
Senior Lecturer in Periodontology

Ken Hemmings
Consultant

John Hobkirk
Professor

Ruth Holt
Senior Lecturer

Elisabeth Horrocks
Consultant

Nigel Hunt
Professor of Orthodontics

Steven Jones
Consultant

Howard Moseley
Consultant

Joseph Noar
Consultant

Stephen Porter
Professor of Oral Medicine

Graham Roberts
Professor of Paediatric Dentistry

Crispian Scully
Dean, Director of Studies and Research

Rosemary Shotts
Honorary Lecturer

Maurizio Tonetti
Professor of Periodontology

all at Eastman Dental Institute for Oral Health Care Sciences, University College London, University of London

Preface

This book gives an overview of oral health and disease and includes summaries of preventive care. Oral lesions may cause considerable pain and loss of quality of life and can also herald local or systemic disease. Some oral lesions, particularly oral cancer, are life-threatening and others mark systemic disease, such as HIV/AIDS. Indeed, the mouth is often a mirror of internal disease.

Patients with oral lesions seek attention and advice from medical, dental, nursing, and pharmaceutical professionals and therefore a concise summary of the aetiology, clinical features, diagnosis and management of the more common lesions, together with references or further reading, should be helpful to these professionals. This book should prove useful to those in medicine, especially general practitioners, dermatologists, internists, paediatricians, oral and maxillofacial surgeons, and otorhinolaryngologists; to those in dentistry, especially oral medicine and pathology, paediatric dentistry, and general practitioners; and also to professionals in nursing and pharmacy.

Detail is included where the lesions are localised to the mouth, or where the oral lesions are pathognomonic or prominent features of the condition. Where oral lesions tend to be a more minor component of the disorder, essential facts only are included.

The book is written with clinical colleagues from the Eastman Dental Institute for Oral Health Care Sciences in London, with advcie from Dr Rosemary Toy (General Practitioner, Rickmansworth, Herts) and other medical and dental colleagues, mainly those at the John Radcliffe Hospital, Oxford, and the Nuffield Orthopaedic Centre, Oxford. We are also grateful to colleagues who have either helped with patient care or provided some of the illustrations.

Professor Crispian Scully CBE

1 Oral health and disease

Ruth Holt, Graham Roberts, Crispian Scully

A healthy dentition and mouth is important to both quality of life and nutrition, and oral disease may affect systemic health, as discussed in later chapters.

Development of the dentition

Teeth form mainly from neuroectoderm and comprise a crown of insensitive enamel surrounding sensitive dentine and a root that has no enamel covering. Teeth contain a vital pulp (nerve) and are supported by the periodontal ligament, through which roots are attached into sockets in the alveolar bone of the jaws (maxilla and mandible). The fibres of the periodontal ligament attach through cementum to the dentine surface. The alveolus is covered by the gingivae, or gums, which, when healthy, are pink, stippled, and tightly bound down and form a close fitting cuff with a small sulcus (gingival crevice) round the neck (cervical margin) of each tooth.

The primary (deciduous or milk) dentition comprises four incisors, two canines, and four molars in each jaw (total of 20 teeth). The normal permanent (adult) dentition comprises four incisors, two canines, four premolars, and six molars in each jaw (32 teeth).

Tooth development begins in the fetus, at about 28 days in utero. Indeed, all the primary and some of the permanent dentition start to develop in the fetus. Mineralisation of the primary dentition begins at about 14 weeks in utero, and all primary teeth are mineralising by birth. The permanent incisors and first molars begin to mineralise at or close to the time of birth, while the other permanent teeth start to mineralise later. Tooth eruption occurs after formation and mineralisation of the crown are largely complete but before the roots are fully formed.

Neonatal teeth are uncommon and may be loose. They may damage the mother's nipple during suckling, in which case they might need to be removed.

- **Tooth development begins in utero**
- **Root formation finalises after eruption**
- **Full primary dentition has 20 teeth**
- **Full permanent dentition has 32 teeth**

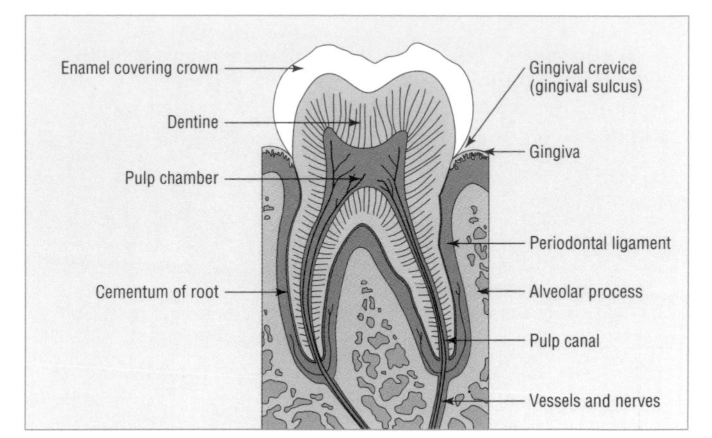

Diagram of a tooth and supporting structures

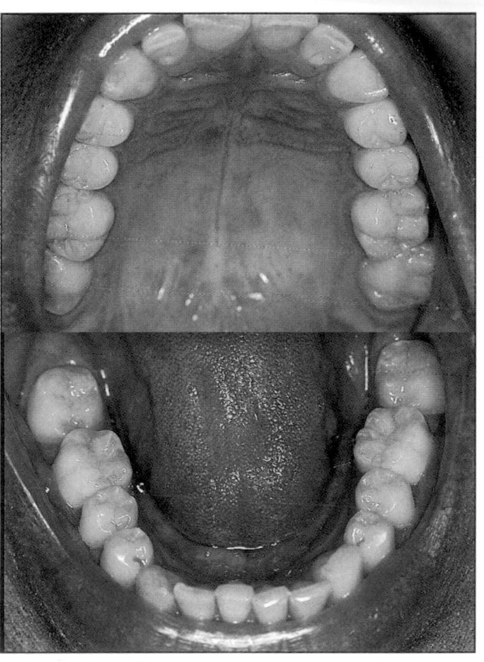

Healthy dentition, increasingly seen as caries declines

Average times of tooth eruption

	Upper teeth	Lower teeth
Primary teeth		
Central incisors	8-13 months	6-10 months
Lateral incisors	8-13 months	10-16 months
Canines (cuspids)	16-23 months	16-23 months
First molars	13-19 months	13-19 months
Second molars	25-33 months	23-31 months
Permanent teeth		
Central incisors	7-8 years	6-7 years
Lateral incisors	8-9 years	7-8 years
Canines (cuspids)	11-12 years	9-10 years
First premolars (bicuspids)	10-11 years	10-12 years
Second premolars (bicuspids)	10-12 years	11-12 years
First molars	6-7 years	6-7 years
Second molars	12-13 years	11-13 years
Third molars	17-21 years	17-21 years

Teething

Eruption of primary teeth may be preceded by a bluish gingival swelling, usually a result of a transient haematoma and, rarely, an eruption cyst, which usually ruptures spontaneously. Tooth eruption may be associated with irritability, disturbed sleep, cheek flushing, drooling, and sometimes a small rise in temperature or a circumoral rash, but it does not cause diarrhoea or bronchitis (although these may occur coincidentally).

Delays in tooth eruption

A delay in eruption of up to 12 months may be of little or no importance in an otherwise healthy child. Localised delays often result from local factors such as a tooth in the path of eruption, insufficient space in the dental arch, or dental infection. Ectopic positioning and impaction most often affect the third molars, second premolars, and canines, possibly because these are the last teeth to erupt.

More generalised failure of eruption is rare but may be associated with a variety of systemic causes.

- **Teething may cause irritability, drooling, and a small rise in body temperature**
- **Failed eruption of single teeth is often caused by impaction**

Causes of delayed tooth eruption

Local
- Impacted teeth

Iatrogenic
- Cytotoxic therapy
- Radiotherapy

Uncommon or rare systemic causes
- Down's syndrome
- Cleidocranial dysplasia
- Congenital hypopituitarism
- Congenital hypothyroidism
- Gaucher's disease
- Osteopetrosis

Early loss of teeth

Early tooth loss is usually because of extraction as a result of dental caries or, in adults, periodontal disease. Teeth, particularly incisors, may also be lost through trauma, such as from sports, assaults, or other injuries.

Unexplained early tooth loss in children or adults may be a feature of Down's syndrome, diabetes, immune defects, or non-accidental injury, or of rare conditions such as eosinophilic granuloma, hypophosphatasia, or Papillon-Lefèvre syndrome (palmoplantar hyperkeratosis).

- **Most tooth loss is due to caries, periodontal disease, or trauma**
- **Early tooth loss may have a systemic cause**

Main causes of early loss of teeth

Local causes
- Caries
- Periodontal disease
- Trauma

Systemic causes	Main systemic features
Genetic defects	
Down's syndrome	Learning disability, short stature
Papillon-Lefèvre syndrome	Palmar-plantar hyperkeratosis
Juvenile periodontitis and related disorders	Sometimes neutrophil defects
Ehlers-Danlos syndrome type VIII	Hypermobility
Chédiak-Higashi syndrome	Recurrent infections
Eosinophilic granuloma	Bone lesions
Immune defects	
Neutropenia	Recurrent infections
Neutrophil defects	Recurrent infections
Monocyte defects	Recurrent infections
Interleukin 1 abnormalities	Recurrent infections
HIV infection and AIDS	Recurrent infections
Enzyme defects	
Acatalasia (absent catalase)	Recurrent infections
Hypophosphatasia (low alkaline phosphatase)	Recurrent infections

Variations in tooth number

Teeth missing from the normal series may have failed to develop (hypodontia) or to erupt or have been lost prematurely.

Hypodontia is not uncommon and is probably of genetic origin. The teeth most often missing are the third molars, second premolars, and maxillary lateral incisors, and other teeth may be reduced in size. Several teeth may be absent in disorders such as Down's syndrome and ectodermal dysplasia.

Mixed dentition—It is not uncommon to see what seem to be two rows of teeth in the lower incisor region, when permanent teeth erupt before the primary incisors have exfoliated. This is particularly likely when there is inadequate space to accommodate the larger permanent teeth. The situation usually resolves as primary incisors are lost and the mandible grows.

Supplemental teeth—Extra teeth are uncommon. Of unknown cause, they are most often seen in the regions of the maxillary lateral incisors, premolars, and third molars. Additional teeth of abnormal form (supernumerary teeth) are also rare. They are usually small and conical in shape and are seen particularly in the maxillary midline, where they may remain unerupted and may cause a permanent incisor to impact. Additional teeth often occur alone in otherwise healthy individuals but occasionally occur in association with rare disorders such as cleidocranial dysplasia and Gardner's syndrome.

- **Missing teeth may be due to failed eruption, tooth loss, or hypodontia**
- **Hypodontia is genetic and is seen in Down's syndrome and ectodermal dysplasia**
- **Supplemental or supernumerary teeth are genetic and occasionally occur with systemic disorders**

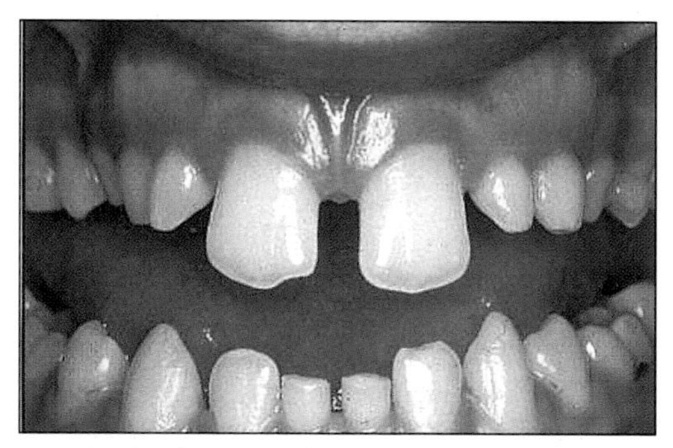

Hypodontia with many missing permanent teeth, including upper lateral incisors and lower central incisors. This appearance may be seen in ectodermal dysplasia

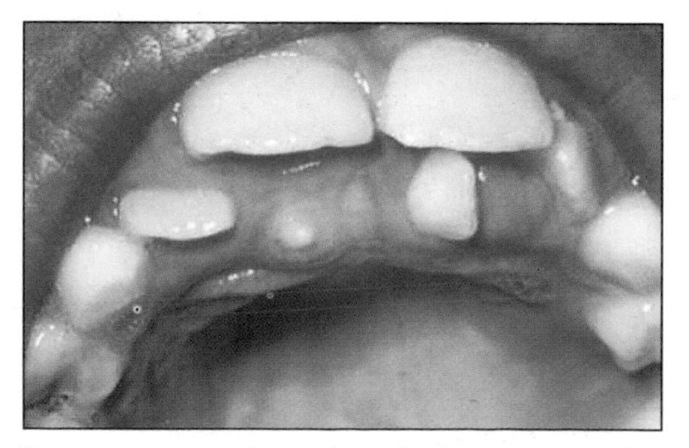

Supernumerary teeth erupting palatal to upper central incisors. Such teeth often remain unerupted and may impede eruption of permanent incisors

Tooth size, shape, structure, and colour

A variety of local and generalised factors may act during tooth formation or mineralisation. Although tooth development in utero is generally well protected, it may be affected by maternal disease and intrauterine infection and by systemic disturbance during early life. Intrauterine infections that may affect tooth structure include rubella and cytomegalovirus. The classic hutchinsonian incisors and Moon's (or mulberry) molars of congenital syphilis are extremely uncommon in developed countries.

Between birth and 6 years of age, the permanent teeth, particularly those of cosmetic importance, may be damaged. Upper permanent incisors may show defects as a consequence of trauma to the primary predecessor. Local infection or trauma may cause a defect in a single tooth or group of teeth. Malformed lower premolars secondary to periapical infection of their primary predecessors are not uncommon and are termed Turner's teeth. More generalised defects may be seen in a range of systemic disorders (prematurity, infections, jaundice, malabsorption, and cytotoxic therapy) during tooth formation and mineralisation, the defect relating to the timing, severity, and duration of the disorder.

Teeth, especially the third molars, may vary in size, form, and structure because of genetic factors. Microdontia (teeth smaller than usual) is largely of genetic origin and usually affects the lateral incisors, which are conical or peg shaped. Teeth that are larger than normal (megadont) are uncommon. Double teeth may be seen occasionally. These seem to be the result of fusion of two teeth and occur most often in the primary dentition, when they are likely to be followed by extra tooth elements in the succeeding permanent dentition.

Superficial tooth discoloration is usually caused by poor oral hygiene or habits such as smoking, consuming certain foods and beverages (such as tea), or taking drugs such as iron, chlorhexidine, or long term oral antimicrobials. In some cultures chewing betel causes staining. Discoloration of a single tooth is usually because the tooth is non-vital, heavily filled, or carious.

Intrinsic staining of a brown or grey colour may be caused by tetracyclines given to pregnant or lactating women or to children under the age of 8 years. Excessive fluoride ingestion during early life may also result in enamel opacities, but, except in those parts of the world where water supplies contain very high levels of fluoride, these are usually extremely mild.

Enamel and dentine defects of genetic origin are rare but are occasionally severe and may take a variety of forms and vary in their inheritance. They can occur in isolation—as amelogenesis imperfecta (defective enamel) or dentinogenesis imperfecta (defective dentine)—or as part of a disorder such as epidermolysis bullosa dystrophica or osteogenesis imperfecta. In some genetic defects of dentine, for example, newly erupted teeth may seem brownish and translucent, an appearance seen in some patients with osteogenesis imperfecta.

- **Developing teeth can be damaged by infection, jaundice, metabolic disorders, drugs, and irradiation**
- **Tetracyclines given to pregnant or lactating mothers, or to children, can discolour teeth**
- **Inherited disorders of enamel or dentine may cause malformation or discoloration**
- **Most tooth discoloration is due to poor oral hygiene, diet, or habits**

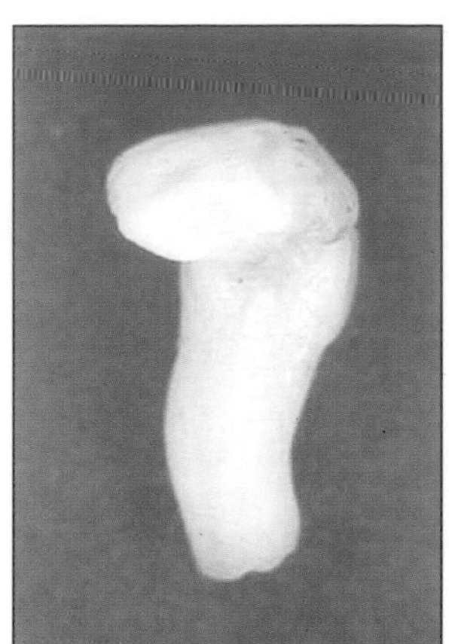

Dilacerated upper central incisor resulting from injury to primary predecessor during permanent tooth development. Severely malformed teeth such as this may require removal, but less severely affected teeth may be treated conservatively

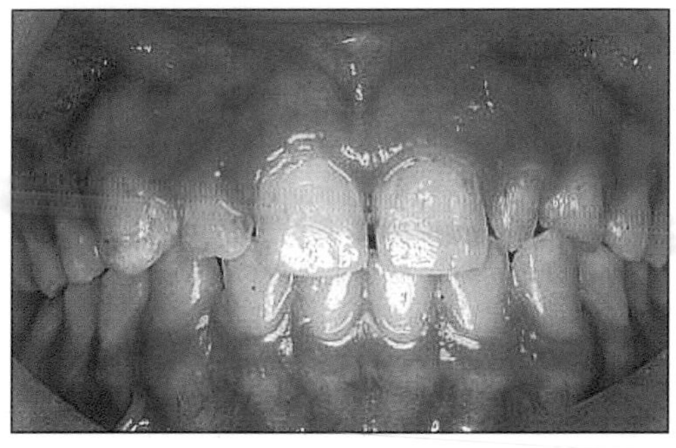

Microdont upper left lateral incisor. The tooth is small in size and conical in form

Causes of tooth discoloration

Extrinsic discolorations (typically brown or black)
- Poor oral hygiene
- Smoking
- Food and drink (such as tea, coffee, red wine)
- Drugs (such as iron, chlorhexidine, antimicrobials)
- Chewing betel

Intrinsic discolorations

Localised
- Trauma (yellow to brown)
- Caries (white, brown, or black)
- Restorative materials (such as black of amalgam)
- Internal resorption (pink spot)

Generalised
- Tetracyclines (brown)
- Excessive fluoride (white or brown)
- Rare causes
  Amelogenesis imperfecta (brown)
  Dentinogenesis imperfecta (brown or purple)
  Kernicterus or biliary atresia (green)
  Porphyria (red)

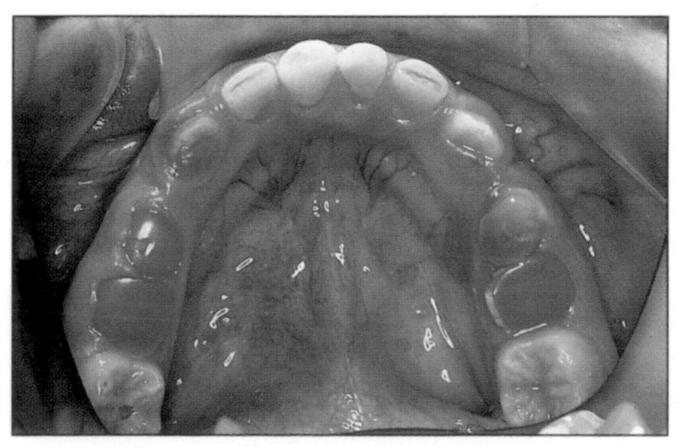

Characteristic appearance of teeth of patient with osteogenesis imperfecta who also shows dentinogenesis imperfecta

Anatomical variants

Patients sometimes become concerned after noticing various anatomical variants in the mouth.

Tori and exostoses are bony lumps that appear during tooth development and are especially common in Mongoloid and Negroid races. Torus mandibularis consists of bilateral, asymptomatic, benign bony lumps lingual to the lower premolars. Also common is torus palatinus, a slow growing, asymptomatic, benign bony lump in the midline of the palate. These lumps are usually left alone but are occasionally excised or reduced if they cause severe difficulties with dentures.

Sebaceous glands may be seen as creamy-yellow dots (Fordyce spots) along the border between the lip vermilion and the oral mucosa. Probably 50-80% of the population have them, but they are not usually clinically evident until after the age of 3 years, and they increase during puberty and then again in later adult life. They are totally benign, although occasional patients or physicians become concerned about them or misdiagnose them as, for example, thrush or lichen planus. No treatment is indicated other than reassurance.

Foliate papillae—The size and shape of the foliate papillae on the posterolateral margins of the tongue are variable. These papillae occasionally swell if irritated mechanically or if there is an upper respiratory infection. Located at a site with a high predilection for lingual cancer, they may give rise to anxiety about cancer.

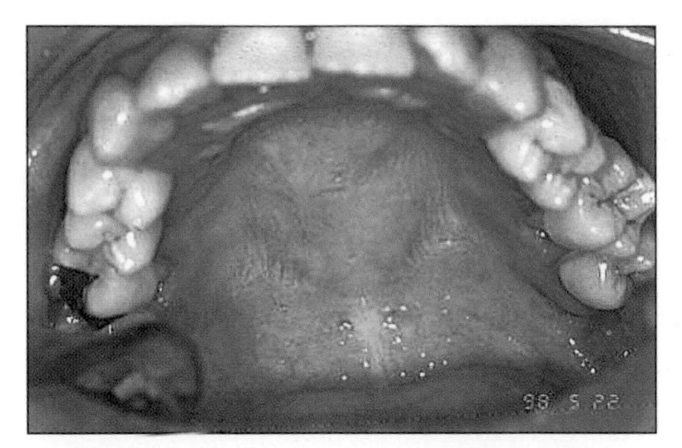

Torus palatinus, with large central torus on palate

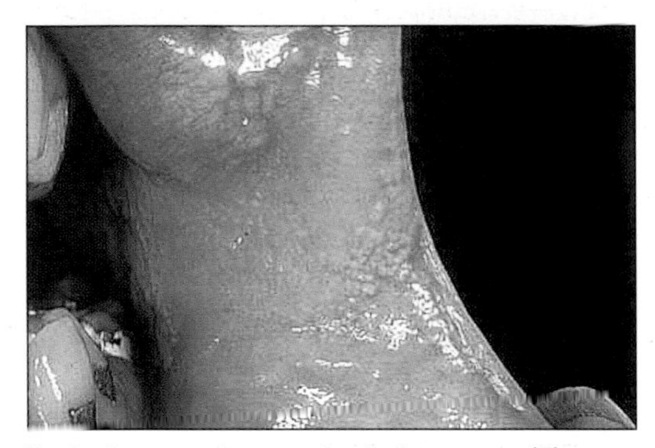

Fordyce's spots—sebaceous glands close to vermillion border between lip and buccal mucosa

Further reading

- Scully C, Flint S, Porter SR. *Oral diseases*. London: Martin Dunitz, 1996
- Scully C, Welbury RA. *Colour atlas of oral diseases in children and adolescents*. London: Mosby Wolfe, 1994

2 Dental damage, sequelae, and prevention

Ruth Holt, Graham Roberts, Crispian Scully

Tooth damage

Teeth may be damaged by dental caries, trauma, erosion, attrition, and abrasion or lost through periodontal disease.

Disease

Caries and inflammatory periodontal disease are the most prevalent oral diseases, both a result of the activity of dental bacterial plaque. Plaque is a complex biofilm containing various microorganisms that forms mainly on teeth and particularly between them, along the gingival margin, and in fissures and pits, adhering by a variety of mechanisms. If plaque is not regularly removed the flora evolves, and plaque may calcify, forming calculus (tartar).

Fermentation of sucrose and other non-milk extrinsic sugars by plaque bacteria to lactic and other acids causes tooth decalcification and, with proteolysis, results in caries (decay). The main causal organism is *Streptococcus mutans*. Caries has been declining for some years, mainly because of the protective effect of fluoride, but it is more prevalent in disadvantaged and deprived people, especially in preschool children.

Accumulation of plaque and a change in the microflora may also cause gingival inflammation (gingivitis). If conditions are appropriate this may progress to damage the periodontal membrane (chronic periodontitis) and lead to tooth loss.

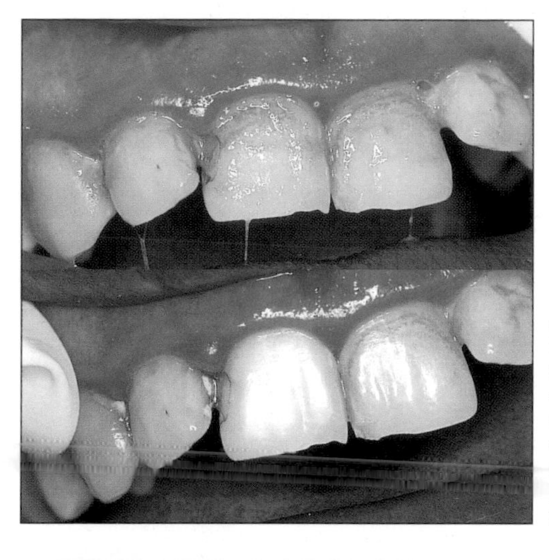

Accumulation of dental plaque close to gingival margins and around the contact areas of teeth (top). Same teeth after brushing (bottom)

• Caries and periodontal disease are the main oral diseases, and dental bacterial plaque underlies these diseases
• Fermentation of sugars by plaque bacteria causes caries by decalcification and proteolysis of enamel and dentine
• Plaque can cause inflammation of the gingiva (gingivitis), and involvement of underlying tissues causes periodontitis

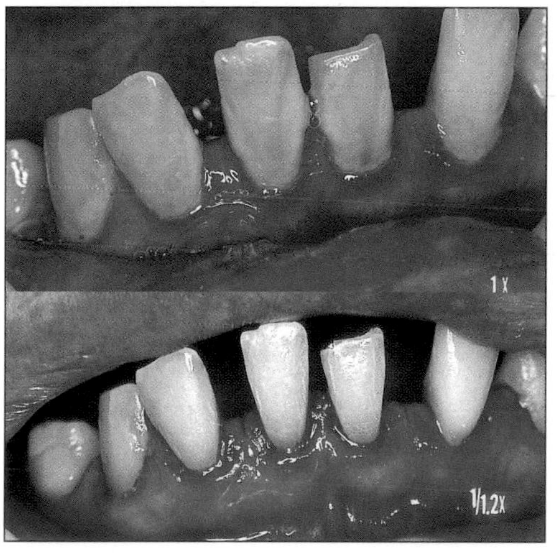

Calculus formed by calcification of plaque (top). Same teeth after calculus removed by scaling (bottom). Calculus cannot be removed by tooth brushing

Other damage

Trauma is common in sport, road accidents, violence, and epilepsy. It occurs mainly in males and usually affects the maxillary incisors.

Tooth erosion is an increasing problem from consumption of carbonated and fruit drinks and occasionally from gastric regurgitation or repeated vomiting (as in bulimia, alcoholism, and gastro-oesophageal reflux). In most cases it results in little more than a loss of normal enamel contour, but in severe cases dentine or pulp may be damaged.

Tooth wear—Attrition, wearing of the biting (occlusal) surfaces, is usually due to tooth grinding (bruxism) or an abrasive diet. Abrasion, wearing at the tooth cervical margin, is mainly caused by brushing with a hard brush or abrasive dentifrice. It can lead to exposure of dentine and therefore sensitivity to hot and cold in particular. Desensitising toothpastes are available, but professional dental care may be needed.

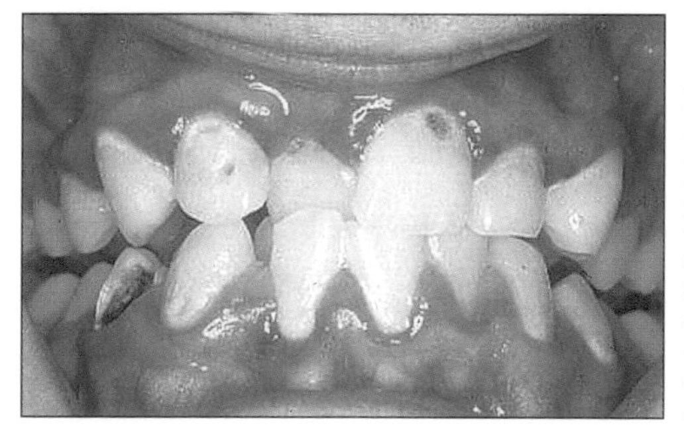

Extensive caries in an adolescent with poor oral hygiene: upper left central incisor and lower right first premolar show obvious caries with large discoloured cavities

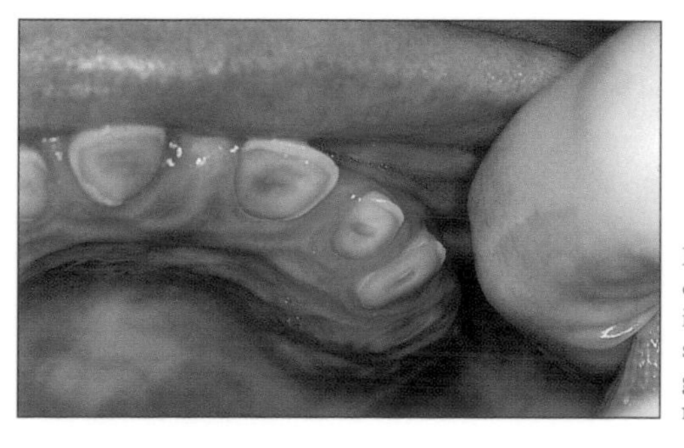

Extreme example of tooth erosion in patient who suffered repeated gastric regurgitation

• Acids readily damage teeth
• Gastric acid or acidic drinks (fruit juices or carbonated drinks) can erode teeth

Sequelae

Most dental pain occurs as a result of caries. Initially, caries presents as a painless white spot (decalcification of the enamel, which may be reversible), followed by cavitation and the appearance of brownish discoloration. Once caries reaches the dentine, pain may result from thermal stimulation or from sweet or sour food or drink. Pain may also occur when dentine is exposed by trauma, erosion, or abrasion; this subsides within seconds of removing the stimulus and may be poorly localised, often only to within two or three teeth of the affected tooth. The tooth should be restored (filled).

Untreated, caries can progress through the dentine to the pulp, which becomes inflamed (pulpitis). Within the rigid confines of the pulp chamber this produces severe persistent pain (toothache), and the pulp eventually undergoes necrosis, when inflammation can spread around the tooth apex (periapical periodontitis), eventually forming an abscess, granuloma, or cyst.

- **Caries in enamel is painless**
- **Caries in dentine may be associated with pain on exposure to heat, cold, or sweet material and if it remains untreated may progress to cause pulpitis**
- **Pulpitis produces severe spontaneous or persistent pain and, if untreated, leads inevitably to pulp necrosis**
- **Pulp necrosis often leads to dental abscess**

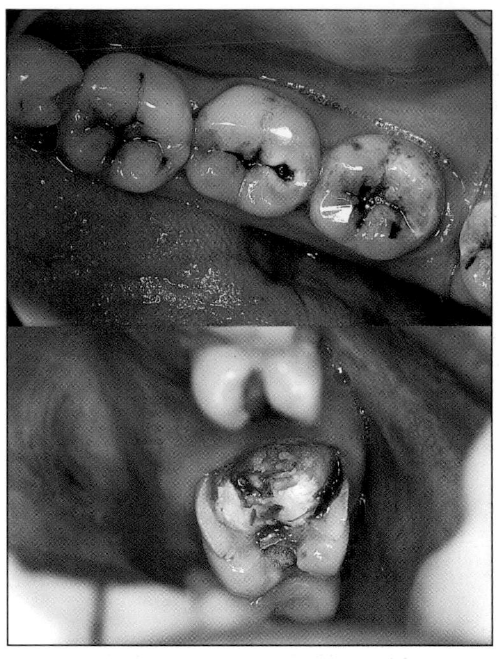

Caries in dentine. Initially, a brown spot with surrounding white area (second molar) is the only outward sign of a large cavity extending into the dentine (top). If untreated, the decay extends to the pulp (red central area, bottom)

Prevention

Diet and lifestyle

Sugars, particularly non-milk sugars in items other than fresh fruits and vegetables, are the major dietary causes of caries. Frequency of intake is more important than the amount.

Dietary advice should start with recommending appropriate infant feeding and weaning practice. Drinks other than milk and water should not be given in feeding bottles and should be confined to main meals. Children should be introduced to a cup at about 6 months of age and should have ceased using bottles by about 1 year. Weaning foods should be free of or very low in sugars other than those present in fresh milk and raw fruits or vegetables.

For older children and adults, snack foods and drinks especially should be free of sugars. Because of the risk of erosion as well as of caries, frequent consumption of carbonated and cola type drinks should be discouraged. Fruit juices can also cause tooth erosion. Water and milk are the preferred options for children.

Saliva buffers may counter plaque acids, and thus chewing sugar-free gum or cheese after meals may be of value. Fresh fruit and vegetables can also confer some protection against oral cancer. However, smoking or chewing tobacco and some other habits may contribute to periodontal disease and oral malignancy, and some chewed products containing sugars may predispose to caries.

Fluorides

Fluorides protect against caries by inhibiting mineral loss, promoting remineralisation of decalcified enamel, and reducing formation of plaque acids. Water fluoridation has consistently been shown to be the most effective, safe, and equitable means of preventing caries and can reduce the prevalence of caries by about half.

Where the water supply contains less than 700 μg/l of fluoride (0.7 ppm), children aged over 6 months who are at high risk of caries may be given daily fluoride supplements as

Four main ways to maintain oral health

Diet
- Reduce consumption and, especially, frequency of intake of food and drink containing sugar
- Food and drink containing sugar should be consumed only as part of a meal
- Snacks and drinks should be free of sugars
- Avoid frequent consumption of acidic drinks

Tooth cleansing
- Brush teeth thoroughly twice daily with a fluoride toothpaste
- Effective plaque removal is essential to prevent periodontal disease
- Tooth brushing alone cannot prevent dental caries, but fluoride toothpastes offer major benefits
- Other aids to plaque removal are a matter for professional advice

Fluoridation
- Request local water company to supply water with optimum fluoride level. Water fluoridation is a safe, equitable, and highly effective public health measure
- Consider use of fluoride supplements for children at high risk and living in areas without water fluoridation

Visiting a dentist
- Have an oral examination every year
- Children and adults at special risk from oral disease, such as those with hyposalivation, or for whom oral disease may be a particular risk to health, such as patients with heart disease, may need more frequent examinations

Modified from *The Scientific Basis of Dental Health Education*; Health Education Authority, 1996

Recommended fluoride dietary supplementation for caries prophylaxis in high risk children in relation to water fluoride content and age

Fluoride in water supply (ppm)*	Child's age			
	<6 months	6 months-3 years	3-6 years	>6 years
<0.3	0	250 μg/day	500 μg/day	1 mg/day
0.3-0.7	0	0	250 μg/day	500 μg/day
>0.7	0	0	0	0

*Local district dental officer or equivalent or water company should be able to supply this information

drops or tablets. However, many toothpastes contain fluoride, which is probably largely responsible for the decline in caries in many countries. Children under about 6 years old may ingest toothpaste, so only a pea sized amount of toothpaste should be used and the brushing supervised in order to reduce the risk of fluorosis (excess fluoride in developing teeth).

Fluoride rinses or gels are useful mainly for patients with special needs or those at high risk of caries, such as people with dry mouths.

Fissure sealants

Plastic coatings placed by a dental professional in the pits and fissures of the permanent teeth can help reduce caries.

Oral hygiene

Good oral hygiene can prevent periodontal disease and oral malodour (halitosis). The most important means of maintaining oral hygiene is using a toothbrush: many types are available, and most are effective at removing plaque. Electric brushes may be useful for those with poor manual dexterity. Tooth brushing at least twice daily with a small headed, medium hardness brush will also help reduce caries if a fluoride toothpaste is used.

However, tooth brushing removes plaque only from smooth dental surfaces and not from the depths of contact areas, pits, and fissures; more effective interdental removal requires regular flossing (some flosses also contain fluoride).

Toothpastes containing triclosan (such as Colgate Total) and chlorhexidine (Corsodyl) have antiplaque activity and have been shown to protect against periodontitis without adverse reactions. Products containing phosphates and phosphonates may help prevent calculus, but some have produced adverse reactions. Many "luxury" toothpastes claim a tooth whitening effect, but few have supporting evidence; distinguishing the results of increased diligence in brushing from a genuine whitening effect of the paste is not straightforward.

Overenthusiastic brushing or an abrasive toothpaste can cause abrasion; silica based toothpastes are less abrasive than those with calcium carbonate or aluminium trihydrate bases.

Mouthwashes are a contentious issue. Many are subject to highly competitive advertising and, although legal constraints ensure that claims are never untrue, the impression gained may be optimistic. Many have only a transient antiseptic activity, some can be harmful by causing mucosal reactions, and they can be dangerous to children, who may ingest them. Most effective antiplaque mouthwashes have prolonged retention on oral surfaces by adsorption and then slow desorption with continued antiplaque activity.

Chlorhexidine helps control plaque and periodontal disease but binds tannins and can thereby cause dental staining if the user drinks coffee, tea, or red wine. This can be cleaned off by dental professionals. Listerine has an antiplaque effect from essential oils and does not stain teeth, but it contains alcohol. Triclosan also has an antiplaque effect.

Vaccination against oral disease

Acceptable, reliably successful vaccines against caries or periodontal disease are not available.

Mouth protection

Soft plastic mouth guards, or occlusal splints, may be needed to prevent damage from trauma, as in sports injuries, or bruxism. For patients with acid reflux, bulimia, or alcoholism, antacids or acid reducing agents may be given to help reduce tooth erosion.

- **Caries and periodontal disease are largely preventable by lifestyle modification**
- **Sucrose and refined carbohydrates are the main causes of caries, and frequency of exposure to these is more important than the total amount consumed**
- **Fluoride reduces caries**
- **Most toothpastes contain fluoride**
- **Fluoride rinses help protect the erupted dentition**
- **Good oral hygiene is essential to prevent gingival and periodontal disease**
- **Tooth brushing twice daily is required for plaque control**
- **Most oral antiseptics have only transient effect**
- **Chlorhexidine, triclosan, and some essential oils have proved antiplaque activity**

Toothpastes accredited by British Dental Association 1999

Normal fluoride
- Macleans Freshmint and Coolmint

High fluoride
- Colgate Triple Cool Stripe
- Colgate Ultra Cavity Protection
- Crest Complete

Low fluoride
- Macleans Milk Teeth
- Macleans Milk Teeth Gel

To reduce sensitivity
- Macleans Sensitive

To reduce gingival disease, caries, tartar
- Colgate Total
- Crest Complete

Whitening
- Macleans Whitening Toothpaste

Antiplaque mouthwashes of proved efficacy

Corsodyl
- Contains chlorhexidine
- May cause tooth staining

Colgate Total Plax*
- Contains triclosan with copolymer

Listerine*
- Contains thymol, eucalyptol, methyl salicylate, menthol
- Contains 26.9% alcohol

*Accredited by the British Dental Association

Further reading

- Murray JJ, ed. *Prevention of oral disease.* Oxford: Oxford University Press, 1996
- Ohrn R, Enzell K, Angmar-Mansson B. Oral status of 81 subjects with eating disorders. *Eur J Oral Sci* 1999;107:157-63
- Scully C, Flint S, Porter SR. *Oral diseases.* London: Martin Dunitz, 1996
- Scully C, Welbury R. *A colour atlas of oral diseases in children and adolescents.* London: Mosby Wolfe, 1994
- Tomar SL, Winn DM. Chewing tobacco use and dental caries among US men. *J Am Dent Assoc* 1999;130:1601-10
- Watt R, Sheiham A. Inequalities in oral health: a review of the evidence and recommendations for action. *Br Dent J* 1999;187:6-12

3 Periodontal disease

John Coventry, Gareth Griffiths, Crispian Scully, Maurizio Tonetti

Most periodontal disease arises from, or is aggravated by, accumulation of plaque, and periodontitis is associated particularly with anaerobes such as *Porphyromonas gingivalis*, *Bacteroides forsythus*, and *Actinobacillus actinomycetemcomitans*. Calculus (tartar) may form from calcification of plaque above or below the gum line, and the plaque that collects on calculus exacerbates the inflammation. The inflammatory reaction is associated with progressive loss of periodontal ligament and alveolar bone and, eventually, with mobility and loss of teeth.

Periodontal diseases are ecogenetic in the sense that, in subjects rendered susceptible by genetic or environmental factors (such as polymorphisms in the gene for interleukin 1, cigarette smoking, immune depression, and diabetes), the infection leads to more rapidly progressive disease. Osteoporosis also seems to have some effect on periodontal bone loss.

The possible effects of periodontal disease on systemic health, via pro-inflammatory cytokines, have been the focus of much attention. Studies to test the strength of associations with atherosclerosis, hypertension, coronary heart disease, cerebrovascular disease, and low birth weight, and any effects on diabetic control, are ongoing.

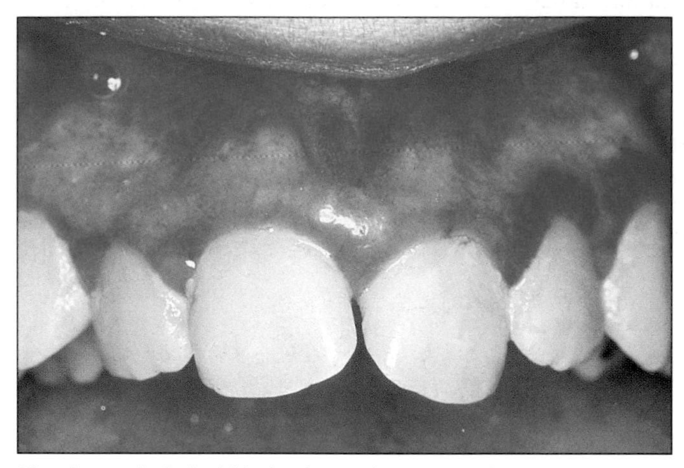

Chronic marginal gingivitis showing erythematous oedematous appearance

Gingivitis

Chronic gingivitis to some degree affects over 90% of the population. If treated, the prognosis is good, but otherwise it may progress to periodontitis and tooth mobility and loss. Marginal gingivitis is painless but may manifest with bleeding from the gingival crevice, particularly when brushing the teeth. The gingival margins are slightly red and swollen, eventually with mild gingival hyperplasia.

Management—Unless plaque is assiduously removed and kept under control by tooth brushing and flossing and, where necessary, by removal of calculus by scaling and polishing by dental staff, the condition will recur. Although gingivitis has a bacterial component, systemic antimicrobials have only transient benefit and therefore no place in treatment. Surgical reduction of hyperplastic tissue by a periodontist (gingivectomy and gingivoplasty) may occasionally be required.

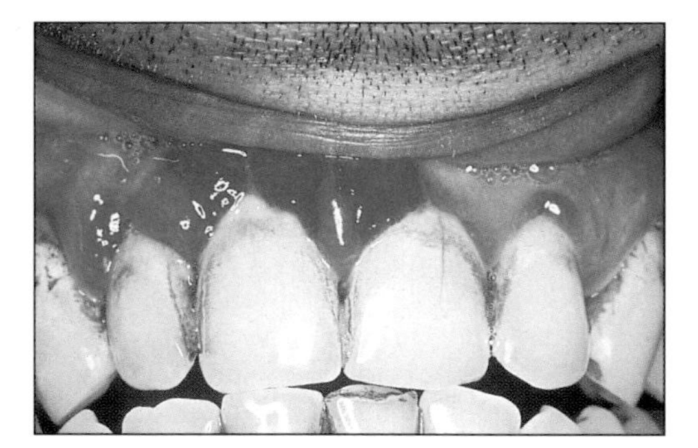

Gingivitis with hyperplasia

- **Good oral hygiene is essential both in preventing and treating periodontal disease**
- **Antimicrobial drugs have no place in treating chronic gingivitis**

Periodontitis

Chronic periodontitis

Chronic periodontitis (inflammation of the gingiva and periodontal membrane) may be a sequel of chronic gingivitis, usually because of accumulation of plaque and calculus. The gingiva detaches from the tooth, the periodontal membrane and alveolar bone are damaged, and an abnormal gap (pocket) develops between the tooth and gum. The tooth may slowly loosen and eventually be lost.

Diagnosis—Chronic periodontitis (pyorrhoea) is typically seen in adults. It is painless but may be associated with bleeding, halitosis, and a foul taste. Debris and pus may be expressed from the pockets, and there may be increasing tooth mobility. Periodontitis cannot be diagnosed by inspection alone, however, and requires specific diagnostic tests (periodontal probing and, sometimes, radiographs).

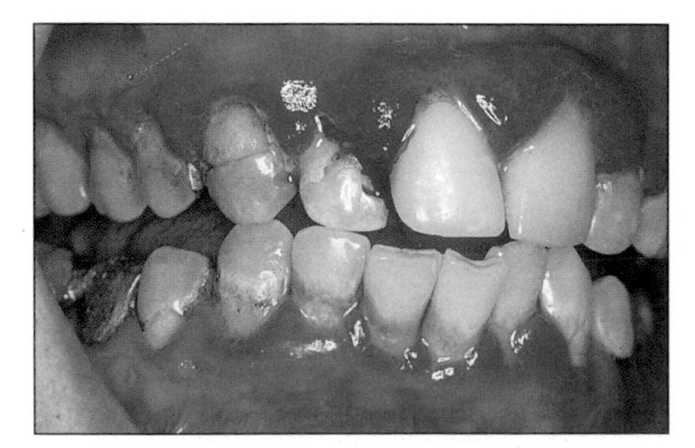

Periodonitis with damage to supporting tissues including bone

Management—Improvement in oral hygiene is necessary, but tooth brushing and mouthwashes have effect only above and slightly below the gum level. They are therefore ineffective in treating periodontitis, as plaque continues to accumulate below the gum line within periodontal pockets. Scaling and polishing and sometimes curettage are also required. Surgical removal of the pocket wall and diseased tissue may be needed to facilitate future cleansing, or attempts to regenerate lost periodontal tissue (such as guided tissue regeneration) may be indicated. Professional attention is therefore required. Although periodontal disease has a bacterial component, systemic antimicrobial drugs have no place in routine treatment, but topical treatment with antimicrobials within the periodontal pockets may be useful.

• Good oral hygiene is essential in treating periodonitis
• Peridonitis requires professional care, usually scaling and polishing and possibly periodontal surgery
• Periodontitis that is unresponsive to such care, advances rapidly, or appears at an early age may have a systemic background

Periodontitis in young patients or which is rapidly advancing
If periodontitis is seen in children or young adults or is rapidly advancing, systemic factors should be excluded.

Gingival bleeding

Bleeding from the gingival margins is common and usually a consequence of gingivitis. It may be more obvious in women taking oral contraceptives and during the second and third trimesters of pregnancy. However, it may be a sign of platelet or vascular disorders and is common in leukaemia and HIV infection.

Causes of gingival bleeding

Local	**Systemic**
• Gingivitis	• Thrombocytopenia
Chronic	Leukaemia
Acute necrotising	HIV infection
• Periodontitis	• Clotting defects
• Rarely, telangiectasia or angioma	Drugs such as anticoagulants

Gingival ulcers

Gingival ulcers are often of infectious aetiology.

Herpes simplex virus stomatitis is common in childhood but is increasingly seen in adults. There is a diffuse, purple, "boggy" gingivitis, especially anteriorly, with multiple vesicles scattered across the oral mucosa and gingiva. This is followed by ulcers. Diagnosis is usually clinical. The infection resolves spontaneously in 7-14 days, during which antipyretic analgesics such as paracetamol and adequate hydration are helpful. Antiviral drugs should be used in severe stomatitis and with immunocompromised patients, who may otherwise suffer severe infection. For those who can safely use it, an aqueous chlorhexidine mouthwash helps to maintain oral hygiene.

Acute necrotising ulcerative gingivitis—Also known as Vincent's disease and trenchmouth, this affects mainly adults and causes painful ulceration of the gums between the teeth (interdental papillae), a pronounced tendency to gingival bleeding, and halitosis. Anaerobic fusiform bacteria and spirochaetes are implicated, and predisposing factors include poor oral hygiene, smoking, malnutrition, and immune defects including HIV and other viral infections and leukaemias. Management includes oral debridement and instruction on oral hygiene, peroxide or perborate mouthwashes, and metronidazole 200 mg three times daily for three days.

Other causes—Gingival ulcers may also be due to aphthae, self injury in psychologically disturbed or mentally challenged patients, malignant neoplasms, drugs, dermatoses, or systemic disease (haematological, mucocutaneous, gastrointestinal, or chronic infections such as tuberculosis, syphilis, mycoses, herpesviruses, and HIV).

• Gingival ulceration in herpetic stomatitis is common and is associated with mouth ulcers elsewhere and fever
• Gingival ulcers with bleeding and halitosis suggest a diagnosis of necrotising gingivitis

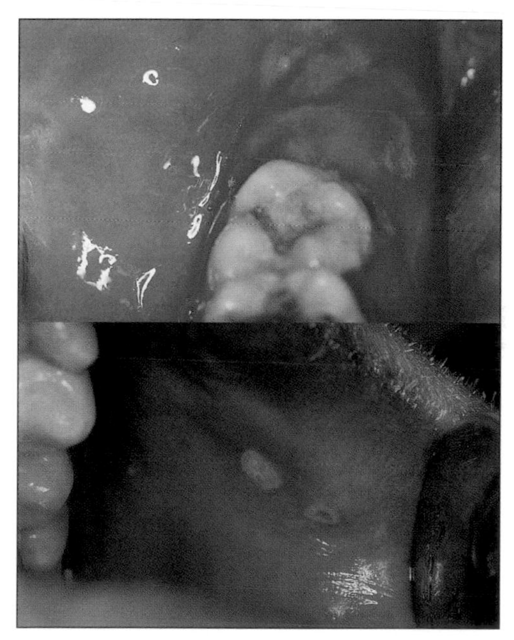

Herpetic stomatitis, with ulcerations on gingivae (top) and elsewhere in the mouth (bottom)

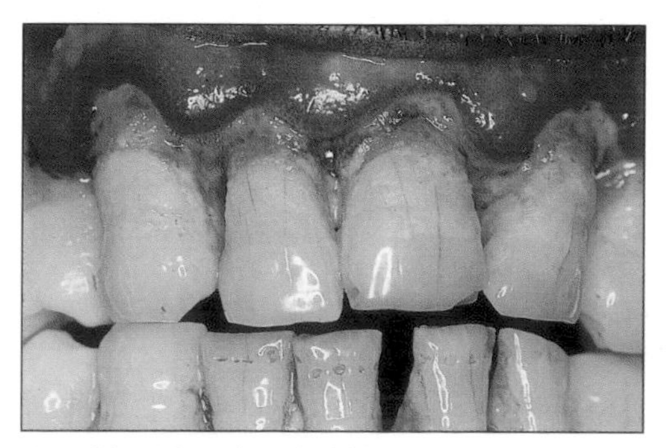

Necrotising (ulcerative) gingivitis

Gingival swelling

Widespread gingival swelling can be a feature of chronic gingivitis and may be caused by drugs, pregnancy, and systemic diseases.

Drug induced gingival swelling—Drugs implicated include phenytoin, cyclosporin, and calcium channel blockers. Gingival swelling is usually worse if there is accumulation of plaque and calculus and the patient is receiving high drug doses. Improved oral hygiene and excision of enlarged tissue may be indicated.

Pregnancy gingivitis—This usually develops around the second month and reaches a peak in the eighth month. An exaggerated inflammatory reaction to plaque in pregnancy predisposes to gingivitis. Oral hygiene should be improved, particularly in view of the current concern that gingivitis may affect fetal birth weight. Pregnancy gingivitis tends to resolve on parturition.

Hereditary gingival fibromatosis—This rare autosomal dominant condition may be associated with hirsutism, but most patients are otherwise perfectly healthy, although there are rare associations with systemic syndromes. Surgical reduction of the gingiva may be indicated.

Causes of gingival swelling

Local causes
- Chronic gingivitis causing
  Gingival abscesses
  Fibrous epulis
- Hyperplastic gingivitis due to mouth breathing causing
  Exostoses
  Cysts
  Pyogenic granuloma
  Neoplasms

Systemic causes
- Hereditary gingival fibromatosis and related disorders
- Drugs (phenytoin, cyclosporin, calcium channel blockers)
- Pregnancy
- Sarcoidosis
- Crohn's disease
- Leukaemia
- Wegener's granulomatosis
- Rarely, amyloidosis, scurvy, midline lethal granuloma, mucopolysaccharidoses, mucolipidoses

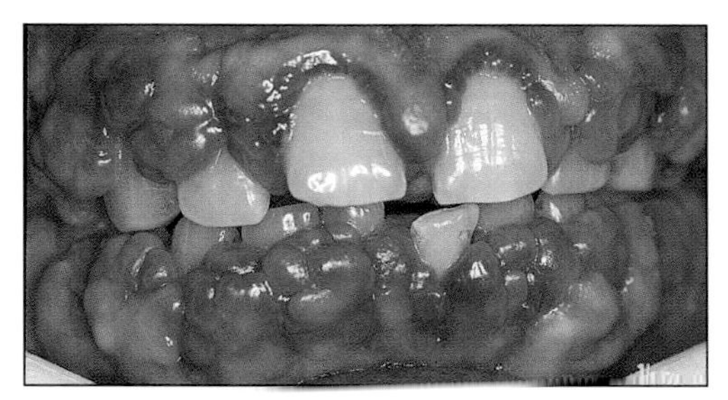

Cyclosporin induced gingival swelling

- **Gingival swelling may occur in pregnancy and typically resolves at parturition**
- **Gingival swelling may be drug induced—by phenytoin, cyclosporin, or calcium channel blockers**

Gingival lumps

Erupting teeth, particularly mandibular third molars, may be associated with swelling and tenderness of the overlying soft tissue flap (operculum), especially if this is traumatised by a tooth in the opposing dental arch. This condition, termed pericoronitis, is best treated by cleaning the area and having a dentist grind or remove the opposing tooth if it is causing trauma. If the patient is in severe pain or is feverish antimicrobials such as metronidazole 200 mg thrice daily for up to five days may be indicated.

Pregnancy epulis—Pregnancy may cause a localised swelling (epulis) of the gingival papillae, which may bleed or ulcerate. Occasionally, a large epulis requires surgical removal.

Fibroepithelial polyp—Also called a fibrous lump and fibrous epulis, this is benign in nature. It may need to be removed.

Malignant causes of gingival lumps include carcinoma, Kaposi's sarcoma, and lymphoma.

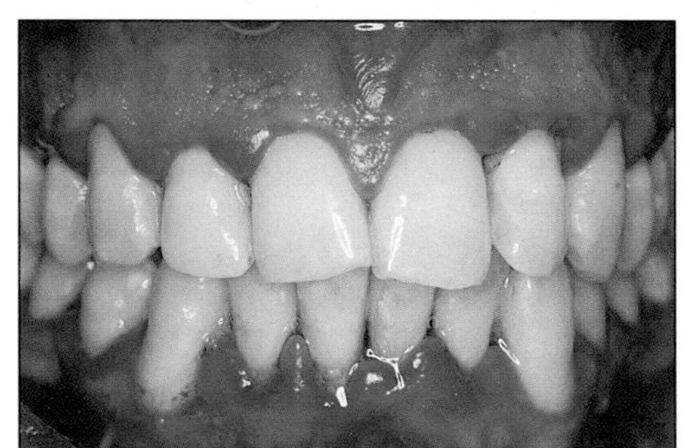

Pregnancy gingivitis

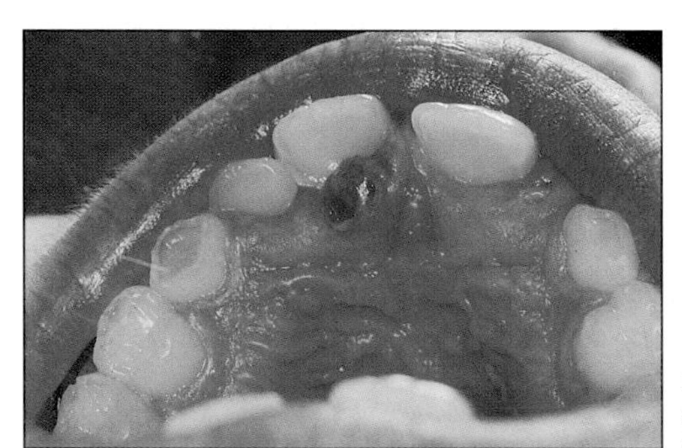

Pyogenic granuloma in a child

Red gingival lesions

The most common cause of redness is gingivitis, in which the erythema is usually restricted to the gingival margins and interdental papillae (see above). Red lesions may also be due to desquamative gingivitis, erythroplasia, haemangiomas, orofacial granulomatosis, Crohn's disease, sarcoidosis, Wegener's granulomatosis, and neoplasms such as carcinoma and Kaposi's sarcoma.

Desquamative gingivitis

Widespread erythema, particularly if associated with soreness, is usually caused by desquamative gingivitis. This is fairly common, is seen almost exclusively in women over middle age, and is usually a manifestation of lichen planus or mucous membrane pemphigoid. Its main features include persistent gingival soreness that is worse on eating and red gingivae. Diagnosis is usually obvious from the history and clinical

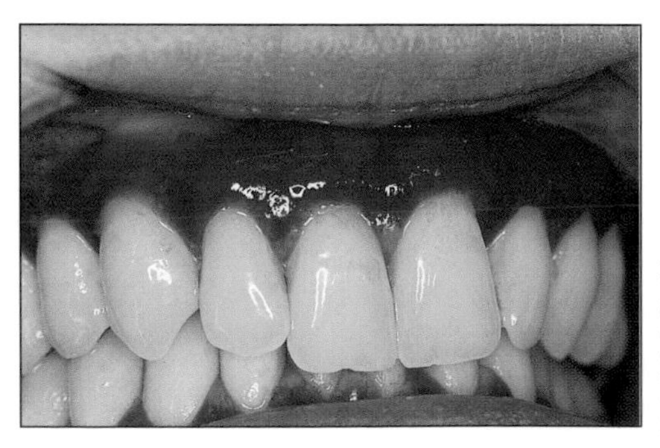

Desquamative gingivitis; usually a sign of pemphigoid (as here) or lichen planus

features, but biopsy and immunostaining may be needed to establish the precise cause.

Management is based on treating the underlying condition and, if there are extraoral lesions, systemic treatment, usually with corticosteroids. Desquamative gingivitis can also often be improved with better oral hygiene and topical corticosteroids such as fluocinonide cream used by a dentist in a plastic splint over the teeth and gums.

• Desquamative gingivitis is not uncommon in women over middle age
• Most desquamative gingivitis is caused by lichen planus or pemphigoid

Gingival pigmentation

This is usually a normal condition mainly seen in certain races (such as black people). Other causes include particles of dental amalgam embedded in the soft tissues, Addison's disease, Kaposi's sarcoma, drugs such as minocycline, melanotic macules and naevi, and melanoma.

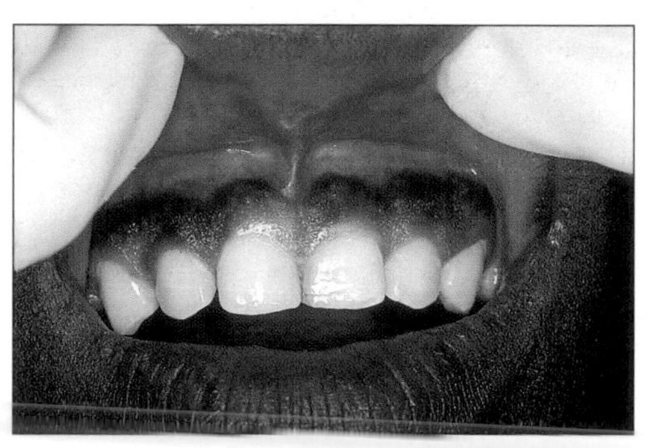

Gingival pigmentation is common in black people

Halitosis

Oral malodour (foetor oris) predominantly originates from the tongue coating, gingival crevice, and periodontal pockets. Plaque organisms—especially *Porphyromonas gingivalis*, fusobacteria, and other anaerobes—cause putrefaction, resulting in release of volatile chemicals, particularly sulphide compounds (including hydrogen sulphide, methylmercaptan, dimethyl sulphide, and dimethyl disulphide).

Some oral malodour is common in healthy individuals, particularly after sleep (morning breath). People who refrain from oral hygiene soon develop malodour, but this is worse with any form of sepsis of the aerodigestive tract such as gingivitis, periodontitis, dental abscess, dry socket, sinusitis, tonsillitis, nasal foreign bodies, and tumours.

Many foods and drinks can cause malodour, especially garlic, onions, curries, the fruit durian, etc. Smoking and drugs—including alcohol, isosorbide dinitrate, and disulphiram—may also be implicated. Rare causes include diabetic ketoacidosis, renal or hepatic dysfunction, and psychiatric disease, as in delusional halitosis or as a feature in schizophrenia.

Management

Management requires establishing the presence of true halitosis and assessing its severity with a portable sulphide monitor (halitometer). Dietary, infective, and systemic causes must be excluded. A full assessment of oral health is always indicated.

The most reliably effective management is

- Improving oral hygiene
- Eating regularly
- Avoiding odiferous foods, drugs, and other substances
- Chewing sugar-free gum regularly
- Using one of the many oral deodorants available over the counter
- Using an antibacterial mouthwash or one such as Retardex or Dentyl
- In severe or recalcitrant cases, using metronidazole 200 mg thrice daily for seven days.

Mouthwashes with antimicrobial activity

Chlorhexidine gluconate
- 0.1-0.2% aqueous mouthwash, rinse for 1 minute twice daily
- Has measurable antiplaque activity
- May stain teeth superficially if patient drinks tea, coffee, or red wine

Povidone iodide
- 1% mouthwash used 2-4 times daily for up to 14 days
- Contraindicated in iodine sensitivity, pregnancy, thyroid disorders, or those taking lithium

Cetypyridinium chloride
- 0.05% mouthwash used twice daily

Hexetidine
- 0.1% mouthwash used twice daily

Further reading

- Beck JD, Pankow J, Tyroler HA, Offenbacher S. Dental infections and atherosclerosis. *Am Heart J* 1999;138:528-33
- Birkenfeld L, Yemini M, Kase NG, Birkenfeld A. Menopause-related oral alveolar bone resorption: a review of relatively unexplored consequences of estrogen deficiency. *Menopause* 1999;6:129-33
- Moore PA, Weyant RJ, Mongelluzzo MB, Myers DE, Rossie K, Guggenheimer J, et al. Type 1 diabetes mellitus and oral health: assessment of periodontal disease. *J Periodontol* 1999;70:409-17
- Morrison HI, Ellison LF, Taylor GW. Periodontal disease and risk of fatal coronary heart and cerebrovascular diseases. *J Cardiovasc Risk* 1999;6:7-11
- Offenbacher S, Beck JD, Lieff S, Slade G. Role of periodontitis in systemic health: spontaneous preterm birth. *J Dent Educ* 1998;62:852-8
- Schenkein H, Committee on Research, Science and Therapy of the American Academy of Periodontology. The pathogenesis of periodontal diseases. *J Periodontol* 1999;70:457-70
- Scully C, Flint S, Porter SR. *Oral diseases*. London: Martin Dunitz, 1996
- Scully C. Oral medicine and periodontology. *Periodontol 2000* 1998;18:7-110

4 Oral cancer

Crispian Scully, Stephen Porter

Most mouth cancer is oral squamous cell carcinoma. This is uncommon in the developed world, except in parts of France, but is common in the developing world, particularly South East Asia and Brazil. It is mainly seen in men over middle age (though it is increasing in younger people), tobacco users, and lower socioeconomic groups.

Aetiological factors (acting on a genetically susceptible individual) include tobacco use (75% of people with oral cancer smoke), betel use (Bidi leaf, and often tobacco, plus spices, slaked lime, and areca nut), alcohol consumption, a diet poor in fresh fruit and vegetables, infective agents (*Candida*, viruses), immune deficiency, and (in the case of lip carcinoma) exposure to sunlight.

Additional primary neoplasms may arise mainly in the aerodigestive tract. This occurs in up to 25% of people who have had oral cancer for over three years, and in up to 40% of those who continue to smoke. Similarly, patients with lung cancer are at risk from second primary oral cancers.

Potentially malignant lesions or conditions may include some erythroplasias, dysplastic leucoplakias (about half of oral carcinomas have associated leucoplakia), lichen planus, submucous fibrosis, and chronic immunosuppression. Rare causes of oral cancer include tertiary syphilis, discoid lupus erythematosus, dyskeratosis congenita, and Plummer-Vinson syndrome (iron deficiency and dysphagia).

• Oral squamous cell carcinoma is mainly a disease of men over middle age, but its prevalence is increasing
• Tobacco use and alcohol consumption are the main aetiological factors
• Patients are at risk from second primary neoplasms

Oral malignant neoplasms

Common
- Squamous cell carcinoma

Uncommon
- Malignant salivary gland tumours
- Malignant melanoma
- Lymphomas
- Neoplasms of bone and connective tissue
- Some odontogenic tumours
- Maxillary antral carcinoma (or other neoplasms)
- Metastatic neoplasms (from breast, lung, kidney, stomach, or liver cancer)
- Langerhans' cell histiocytoses
- Kaposi's sarcoma

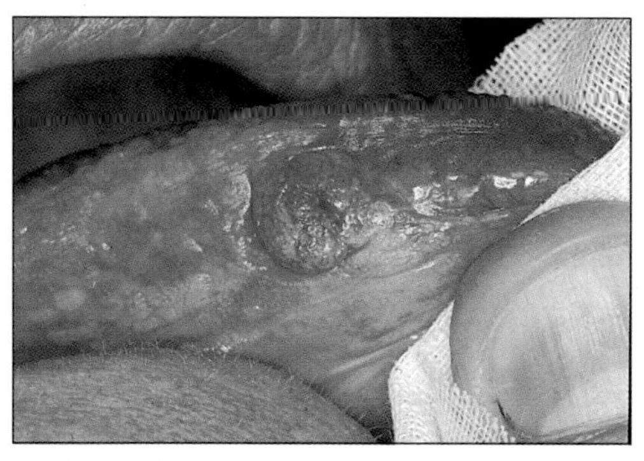

Carcinoma of tongue presenting as a lump

Diagnosis

Too many patients with oral cancer present or are detected late, with advanced disease and lymph node metastases. With earlier detection, treatment is less complicated, the cosmetic and functional results are better, and survival is improved.

Carcinomas may present anywhere in the oral cavity, often on the posterolateral margin of the tongue and floor of the mouth—the "coffin" or "graveyard" area. It is crucial, therefore, not only to examine visually and manually the whole oral cavity but to carefully inspect and palpate the posterolateral margins of the tongue and the floor of the mouth. There is usually a solitary chronic ulceration, red or white lesion, indurated lump, fissure, or enlarged cervical lymph node. Lip carcinoma presents with thickening, crusting, or ulceration, usually of the lower lip.

Enlargement of an anterior cervical lymph node may be detectable by palpation. Some 30% of patients present with palpably enlarged nodes containing metastases, and, of those who do not, a further 25% will develop nodal metastases within two years. Molecular techniques show tumour to be present in many histologically normal nodes.

There should therefore be a high index of suspicion, especially of a solitary lesion present for over three weeks, particularly if it is indurated, there is cervical lymphadenopathy, or the patient is in a high risk group.

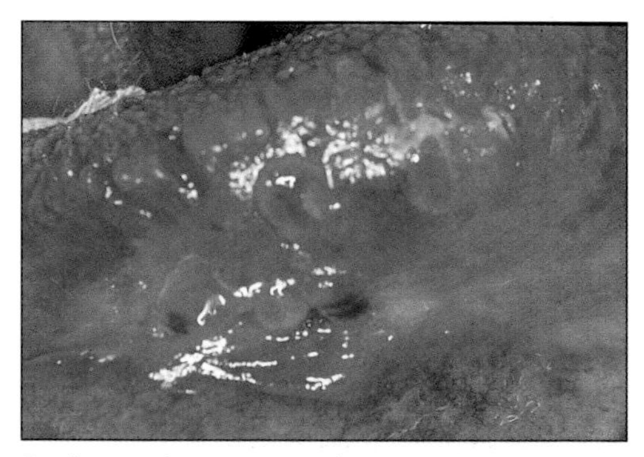

Carcinoma of tongue presenting as an ulcer

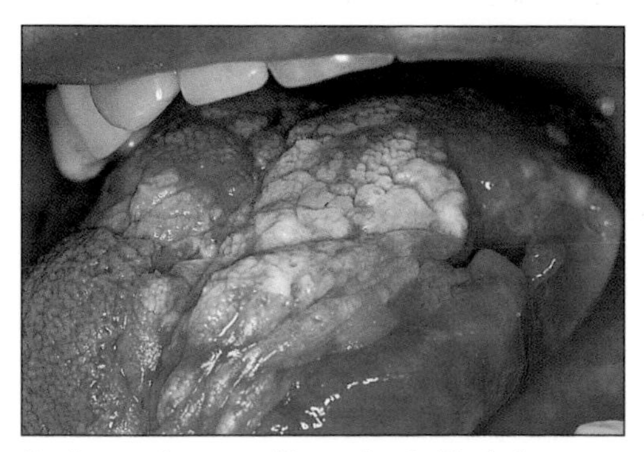

Carcinoma of tongue with associated white lesions

Investigations
It is essential to confirm the diagnosis and determine whether cervical lymph nodes are involved or there are other primary tumours or metastases. Therefore, almost invariably indicated are

- Lesional biopsy (usually an incisional biopsy, but an oral brush biopsy is now available, mainly for cases of widespread potentially malignant lesions and for revealing malignancy in lesions of more benign appearance)
- Jaw and chest radiography
- Endoscopy
- Full blood count and liver function tests.

Computed tomography or magnetic resonance imaging help determine a tumour's extent and invasion, and involvement of the cervical lymph nodes. Ultrasound guided cytology of nodes may help. The staging systems of tumour, nodes, metastases (TNM) classification and T and N integer score (TANIS) are often used. Molecular techniques are being introduced for prognostication in potentially malignant lesions and tumours and to identify nodal metastases.

• Potentially malignant lesions include erythroplasia and some white lesions
• Oral cancer may present as a solitary lump, ulcer, or red or white lesion
• Ealier diagnosis offers better treatment, cosmetic and functional outcome, and survival
• Any oral lesion persisting more than three weeks should be treated with suspicion
• Biopsy is mandatory
• Second primary neoplasms must be excluded

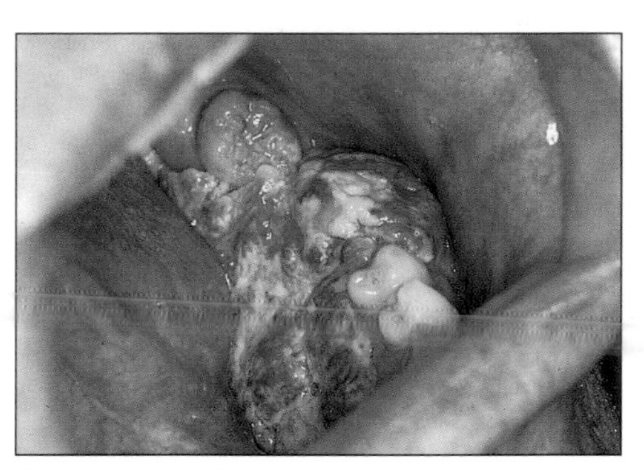

Carcinoma of gingiva

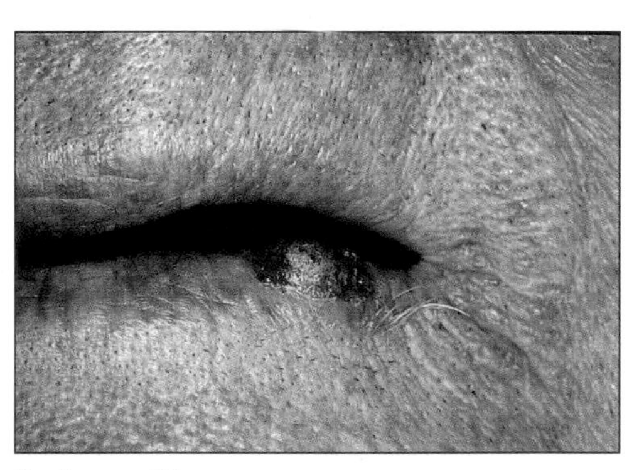

Carcinoma of lip

Management

The prognosis of oral squamous cell carcinoma is very site dependent. For intraoral carcinoma, five year survival may be as low as 30% for posterior lesions presenting late, as they often do. For lip carcinoma, however, five year survival is often over 70%. Important factors to consider in management are quality of life and patient education: in one study, at least six months after the diagnosis of oral cancer, 47% of patients still smoked and 36% drank alcohol to excess. Only a third were aware that these habits were important in the development of oral cancer.

Oral squamous cell carcinoma is now treated largely by surgery or irradiation, although there are few unequivocal controlled trials of treatment modalities. Photodynamic therapy and chemotherapy have occasional applications. Combined clinics, with both surgeons and oncologists, and support staff, usually have an agreed treatment policy and offer the best outcomes.

Surgery

Surgery allows the complete excision of a tumour and lymph nodes and full histological examination for staging, which has implications for prognostication and assessing the need for adjuvant radiotherapy. It can also be used for radioresistant tumours. Disadvantages are mainly the perioperative mortality and morbidity, but modern techniques have significantly decreased these and aesthetic and functional defects.

Patients who succumb to oral cancer almost always die because of failure to control the primary cancer or because of nodal metastases. Death due to distant metastasis is unusual.

Ablative surgery excises the cancer with, ideally, at least a 2 cm margin of clinically normal tissue. If a node has clinical signs of invasion it is reasonable to presume that others may also be involved, and they must be removed by traditional radical neck dissection. "Functional" neck dissections, modified to preserve the jugular, sternomastoid, or accessory nerve while ensuring complete removal of involved nodes, have gained popularity. Moderate dose radiotherapy is sometimes used to "sterilise" such necks.

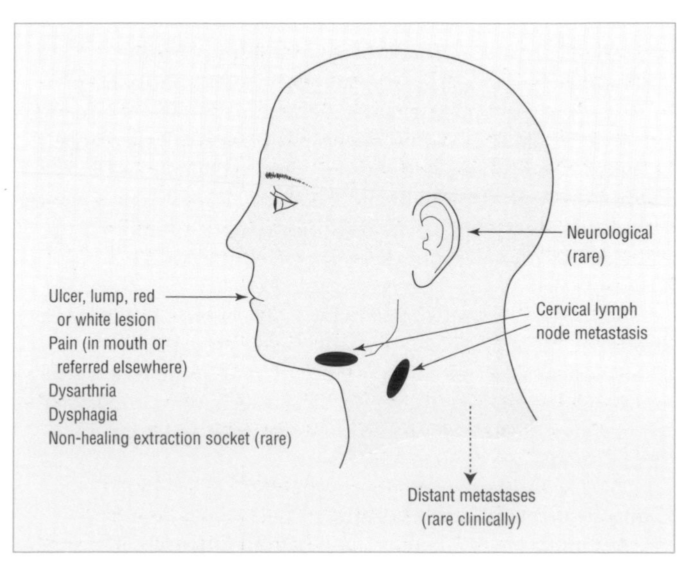

Possible features of oral carcinoma

Reconstruction

Reconstruction is tailored to the patient's ability to cope with a long operation and the risk of substantial morbidity.

Soft tissue reconstruction

Local flaps (such as nasolabial flaps) provide thin reliable flaps suitable for repairing small defects. However, tissue must often be brought into the region in order to repair larger defects. For these, split skin grafts or flaps, free flaps or pedicle flaps, are required.

Free flaps—Microvascular surgery facilitates excellent reconstruction in a single operation by means of, for example, forearm flaps based on radial vessels, which are particularly useful to replace soft tissue. Alternatively, flaps based on the fibula may be used if bone is also required.

Pedicle flaps—Myocutaneous or osteomyocutaneous flaps are based on a feeding vessel to muscle and perforators to the skin paddle. They may be used in a one stage operation to replace skin, and, since they also contain muscle, they have adequate bulk to repair defects and may also be used to import bone (usually rib). Examples include flaps based on the pectoralis major, latissimus dorsi, or trapezius. Flaps from the forehead or deltopectoral pedicle were once the mainstay for reconstruction, but they required a two stage operation, replaced only skin, and relied on a tenuous blood supply.

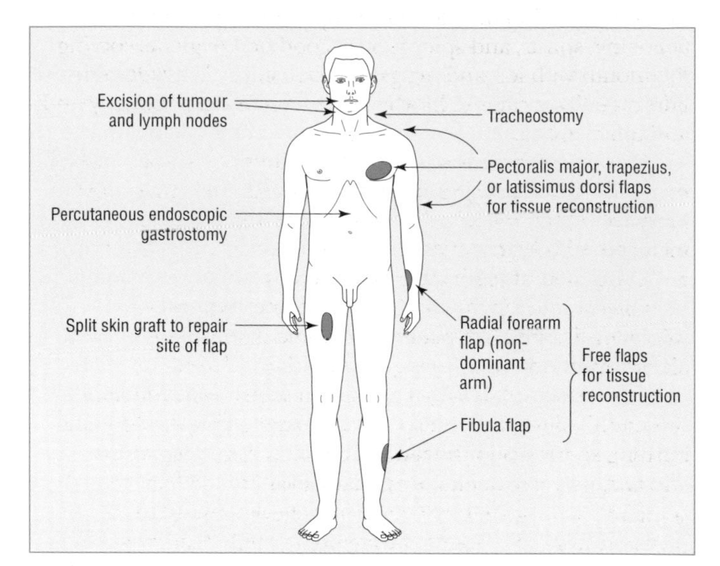

Surgical procedures that may be used in treating patients with oral cancer

Hard tissue reconstruction

Ideally, hard tissue reconstruction is done at the time of tumour resection. Dental implants can then be inserted to carry a prosthesis. Bone is traditionally taken as free non-vascularised bone grafts from iliac crest or rib, but these may survive poorly if contaminated or the vascularity is impaired after irradiation. In such cases, or where there is a large defect, an osteomyocutaneous flap greatly improves the graft's vascular bed. True free vascularised bone grafts such as fibula grafts have great benefits, but they are time consuming and require considerable expertise.

The benefits of bone grafting for maxillary defects are less certain, and maxillary reconstruction is usually with an obturator (bung), which has the advantage that the cavity can be readily inspected subsequently.

Specific complications from the surgery of oral cancer may include infection and rupture of the carotid artery, salivary fistulae, and thoracic duct leakage (chylorrhoea).

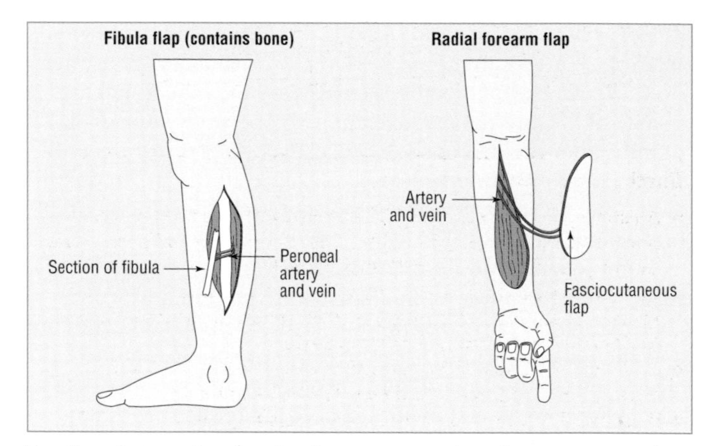

Free flaps that may be taken for tissue reconstruction after tumour resection

Radiotherapy

With radiotherapy, normal anatomy and function are maintained, general anaesthesia is not needed, and salvage surgery is still available if radiotherapy fails. However, adverse effects are common, cure is uncommon (especially for large tumours), and subsequent surgery is more difficult and hazardous (with survival further reduced). Radiotherapy can be delivered by external beams or by implanting a radioisotope.

External beam radiation (teletherapy) is commonly accompanied by side effects (see below).

Interstitial therapy (brachytherapy, plesiotherapy)—Implants of iridium-192 for a few days are often used, giving a radiation dose equivalent to teletherapy but confined to the lesion and immediate area. Plesiotherapy thus causes fewer complications and can be effective, especially for tumours less than 2 cm in diameter and in selected sites.

• Dental treatment, both preventive and curative, is essential before radiotherapy to minimise oral disease and the possible adverse consequences of operative intervention

Complications of radiotherapy

Immediate complications include painful mucositis. The time to healing depends on the radiation dose but is usually

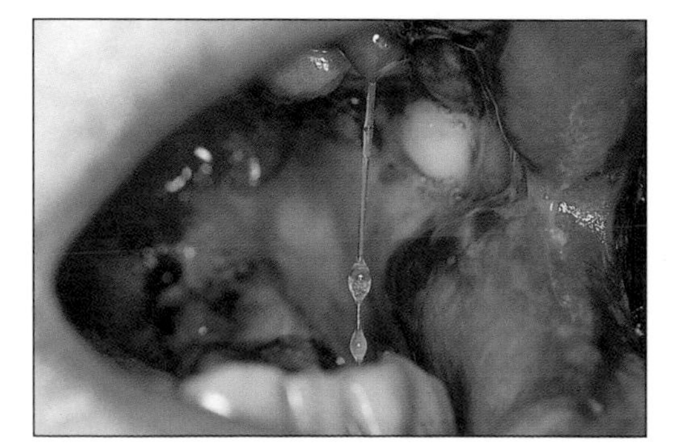

Radiation induced mucositis

complete within three weeks of the end of treatment. Tobacco smoking delays resolution, and mucositis can provide a portal for systemic infection. Mucositis can be reduced by minimising doses of radiation or cytotoxic drugs, avoiding irritants (smoking, spirits, and spicy foods), good oral hygiene, cooling the mouth with ice, and drugs (topical aspirin, benzydamine, lidocaine (lignocaine), chlorhexidine, sucralfate, or polymyxin E and tobramycin).

Osteoradionecrosis is a potentially serious complication. The mandible, with its high density and poor vascularity, is more prone to it than the maxilla. Risk of osteoradionecrosis increases with high radiation dose, fraction size and number, and extraction of teeth after radiotherapy.

Complications in children include enamel hypoplasia, microdontia, impaired tooth development and eruption, and alterations to the developing craniofacial skeleton.

Dry mouth (xerostomia) may cause a subjective complaint of dry mouth, difficulty with speech and swallowing dry foods, a burning sensation in the mouth, dental caries, oral candidiasis, and bacterial sialadenitis. Residual salivary tissue may be stimulatable by gustatory (sugar-free chewing gum) or pharmacological (cholinergic agents) stimuli. Pilocarpine in doses of up to 5 mg three times daily can be effective. Patients with a dry mouth should avoid anything that further impairs salivation—such as drugs, tobacco, and alcohol—and may benefit from frequent sips of water (particularly during eating), saliva substitutes (such as Artificial Saliva, Saliva Orthana, Oralbalance), dietary control, and topical fluorides.

Other complications include loss of taste and cervical atherosclerosis.

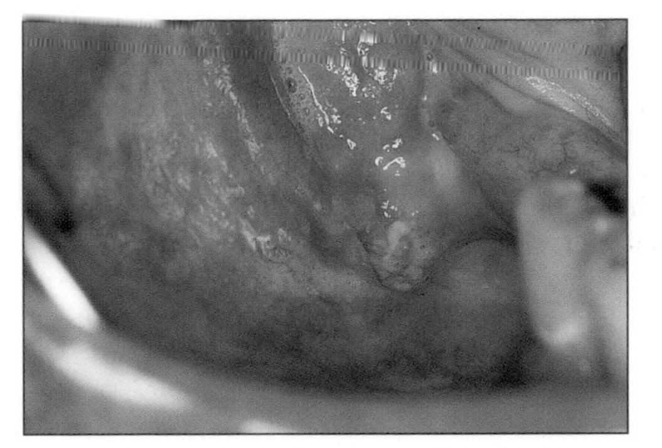

Osteoradionecrosis affecting the mandible, showing exfoliating necrotic bone

Causes of a complaint of dry mouth

Iatrogenic
- Drugs
  Anticholinergics (such as antidepressants, antihistamines, antihypertensives, antiretrovirals)
  Sympathomimetics (such as bronchodilators)
- Irradiation damage
- Graft versus host disease

Salivary gland disease
- Sjögren's syndrome
- HIV infection
- Hepatitis C virus
- HTLV-I infection
- Sarcoidosis
- Aplasia

Dehydration
- Uncontrolled diabetes

Psychogenic

Further reading

- Allison PJ, Locker D, Feine JS. The relationship between dental status and health-related quality of life in upper aerodigestive tract cancer patients. *Oral Oncol* 1999;35:138-43
- Cancer Research Campaign. *Factsheet 14.1.* London. CRC, 1993
- Prince S, Bailey BM. Squamous carcinoma of the tongue: review. *Br J Oral Maxillofac Surg* 1999;37:164-74
- Rodrigues VC, Moss SM, Tuomainen H. Oral cancer in the UK: to screen or not to screen. *Oral Oncol* 1998;34:454-65
- Rogers SN, Hannah L, Lowe D, Magennis P. Quality of life 5-10 years after primary surgery for oral and oro-pharyngeal cancer. *J Craniomaxillofac Surg* 1999;27:187-91
- Schepman K, der Meij E, Smeele L, der Waal I. Concomitant leukoplakia in patients with oral squamous cell carcinoma. *Oral Dis* 1999;5:206-9
- Sciubba JJ. Improving detection of precancerous and cancerous oral lesions. Computer-assisted analysis of the oral brush biopsy. US Collaborative OralCDx Study Group. *J Am Dent Assoc* 1999;130: 1445-57
- Scully C, Ward-Booth P. Detection and treatment of early cancers of the oral cavity. *Crit Rev Oncol Haematol* 1995;21:63-75

5 Mouth ulcers and other causes of orofacial soreness and pain

Crispian Scully, Rosemary Shotts

Ulcerative conditions

Mouth ulcers are common and are usually due to trauma such as from ill fitting dentures, fractured teeth, or fillings. However, patients with an ulcer of over three weeks' duration should be referred for biopsy or other investigations to exclude malignancy (see previous article) or other serious conditions such as chronic infections.

Ulcers related to trauma usually resolve in about a week after removal of the cause and use of benzydamine hydrochloride 0.15% mouthwash or spray (Difflam) to provide symptomatic relief and chlorhexidine 0.2% aqueous mouthwash to maintain good oral hygiene.

• Patients with a mouth ulcer lasting over three weeks should be referred for biopsy or other investigations to exclude malignancy or other serious conditions

Main systemic and iatrogenic causes of oral ulcers

Microbial disease
- Herpetic stomatitis
- Chickenpox
- Herpes zoster
- Hand, foot, and mouth disease
- Herpangina
- Infectious mononucleosis
- HIV infection
- Acute necrotising gingivitis
- Tuberculosis
- Syphilis
- Fungal infections

Cutaneous disease
- Lichen planus
- Pemphigus
- Pemphigoid
- Erythema multiforme
- Dermatitis herpetiformis
- Linear IgA disease
- Epidermolysis bullosa
- Chronic ulcerative stomatitis
- Other dermatoses

Malignant neoplasms

Blood disorders
- Anaemia
- Leukaemia
- Neutropenia
- Other white cell dyscrasias

Gastrointestinal disease
- Coeliac disease
- Crohn's disease
- Ulcerative colitis

Rheumatoid diseases
- Lupus erythematosus
- Behcet's syndrome
- Sweet's syndrome
- Reiter's disease

Drugs
- Cytotoxic agents
- Nicorandil
- Others

Radiotherapy

Recurrent aphthous stomatitis (aphthae, canker sores)
Recurrent aphthous stomatitis typically starts in childhood or adolescence with recurrent small, round, or ovoid ulcers with circumscribed margins, erythematous haloes, and yellow or grey floors. It affects at least 20% of the population, and its natural course is one of eventual remission. There are three main clinical types:
- Minor aphthous ulcers (80% of all aphthae) are less than 5 mm in diameter and heal in 7-14 days
- Major aphthous ulcers are large ulcers that heal slowly over weeks or months with scarring
- Herpetiform ulcers are multiple pinpoint ulcers that heal within about a month.

Some cases have a familial and genetic basis, but most patients seem to be otherwise well. However, a minority have aetiological factors that can be identified, including stress, trauma, stopping smoking, menstruation, and food allergy.

Aphthae are also seen in haematinic deficiency (iron, folate, or vitamin B-12); coeliac disease; Crohn's disease; HIV infection, neutropenia, and other immunodeficiencies; Neumann's bipolar aphthosis, where genital ulcers may also be present; and Behcet's syndrome, where there may be genital, cutaneous, ocular, and other lesions. The mouth ulcers in Behcet's syndrome are often major aphthae with frequent episodes and long duration to healing.

In children aphthae also occur in periodic fever, aphthous stomatitis, pharyngitis, and cervical adenitis syndrome. This syndrome resolves spontaneously, and long term sequelae are rare. Corticosteroids are highly effective symptomatically; tonsillectomy and cimetidine treatment have been effective in some patients.

Diagnosis of aphthae is based on the patient's history and clinical features since specific tests are unavailable. A full blood picture (haemoglobin concentration, white cell count and differential, and red cell indices), iron studies, and possibly red cell folate and serum vitamin B-12 measurements and other investigations may help exclude systemic disorders, which should be suspected if there are features suggestive of a systemic background. Biopsy is rarely indicated.

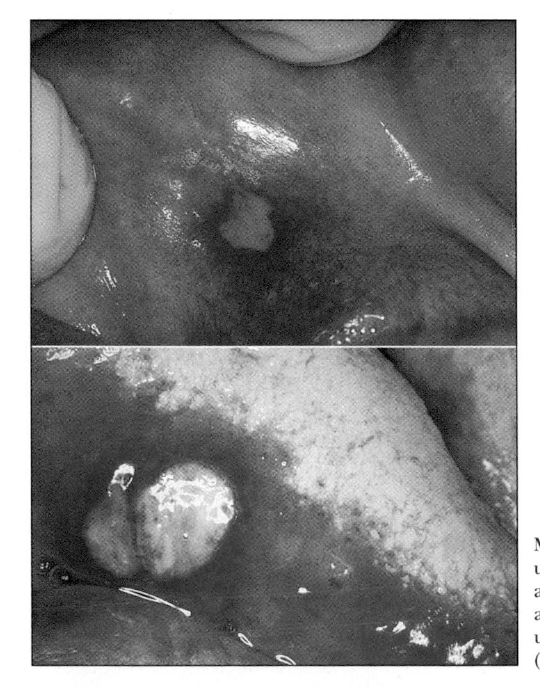

Minor aphthous ulceration (top) and major aphthous ulceration (bottom)

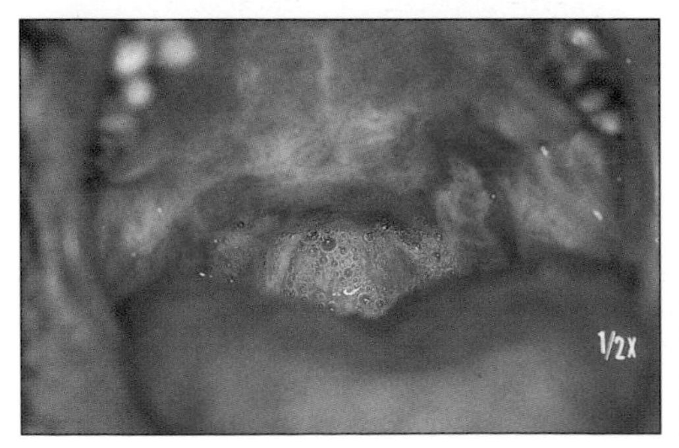

Major aphthous ulceration with severe scarring in patient with Behcet's syndrome

Management Predisposing factors should be identified and corrected. Chlorhexidine mouthwashes may help. Symptoms can often be controlled with hydrocortisone hemisuccinate pellets or triamcinolone acetonide in carboxymethyl cellulose paste four times daily, but more potent topical corticosteroids may be required. Systemic corticosteroids are best given by a specialist. Thalidomide is also effective but is rarely indicated.

Malignant ulcers
Oral carcinoma may present as a solitary chronic ulceration (see previous article).

Mouth ulcers in systemic disease
Ulcers may be manifestations of disorders of skin, connective tissue, blood, or gastrointestinal tract.

The main skin disorders are lichen planus, pemphigus, pemphigoid, erythema multiforme, epidermolysis bullosa, and angina bullosa haemorrhagica (blood filled blisters that leave ulcerated areas after rupture). In view of the clinical consequences of pemphigus, accurate diagnosis of oral bullae is important, and referral for direct and indirect immunofluorescence of biopsy tissue is often indicated.

Drug induced mouth ulcers
Among the drugs that may be responsible for mouth ulcers are cytotoxic agents, antithyroid drugs, and nicorandil.

Non-ulcerative causes of oral soreness

Erythema migrans (benign migratory glossitis, geographic tongue)
This common condition of unknown aetiology, which affects about 10% of children and adults, is characterised by map-like red areas of atrophy of filiform tongue papillae in patterns that change even within hours. The tongue is often fissured. Lesions can cause soreness or may be asymptomatic.

Management—There is no reliably effective treatment, although some have reported efficacy for zinc supplements. Similar lesions may be seen in Reiter's syndrome and psoriasis.

Burning mouth syndrome (oral dysaesthesia, glossopyrosis, glossodynia)
This condition is common in people past middle age and is characterised by a persistent burning sensation in the tongue, usually bilaterally. The cause is unclear, but response to topical anaesthesia suggests it is a form of neuropathy. Discomfort is sometimes relieved by eating and drinking, in contrast to the pain from ulcerative lesions, which is typically aggravated by eating.

Organic causes of discomfort—such as erythema migrans, lichen planus, a deficiency glossitis (related to deficiency of iron, folate, or vitamin B-12), xerostomia, diabetes, and candidiasis—must be excluded, but these are only occasional causes. More often there is an underlying depression, monosymptomatic hypochondriasis, or anxiety about cancer or a sexually transmitted disease. Burning mouth syndrome is more common in Parkinson's disease.

Management—Reassurance and occasionally psychiatric consultation, vitamins, or antidepressants may be indicated, but they are not reliably effective.

Desquamative gingivitis
Widespread erythema, particularly if associated with soreness, is usually caused by desquamative gingivitis. This is fairly common and is seen almost exclusively in women over middle age (see earlier article).

• Patients with aphthae are usually otherwise healthy
• Systemic diseases that should be excluded include Behcet's syndrome, gluten sensitive enteropathy, deficiencies of haematinics, and, occasionally, immunodeficiency
• Recurrent aphthous stomatitis is a clinical diagnosis
• Predisposing factors should be identified and corrected
• Topical corticosteroids aid resolution of ulcers
• In severe cases systemic immunomodulation may be needed

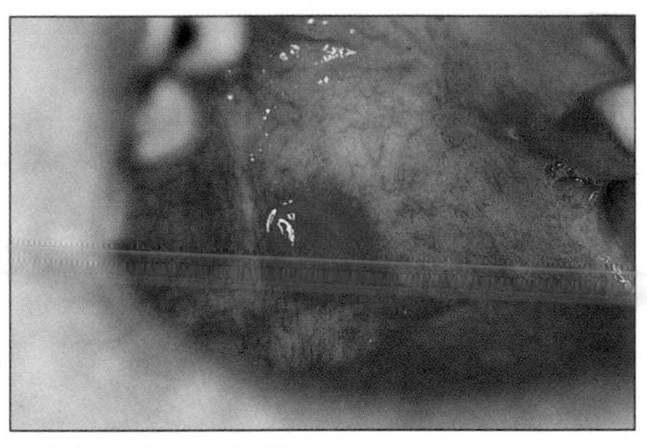

Bulla in oral pemphigoid

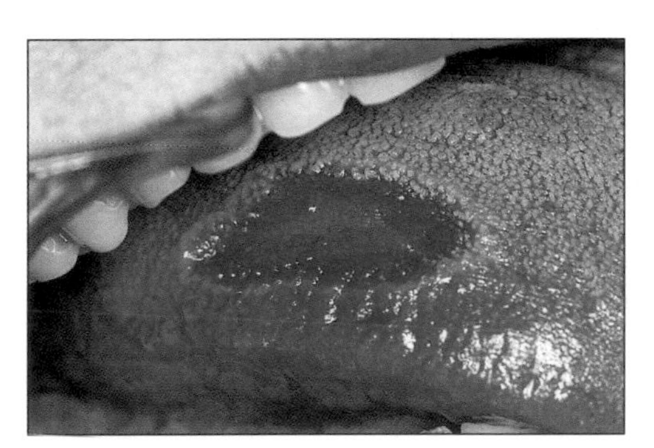

Erythema migrans

Causes of a complaint of burning mouth syndrome

• Local	• Deficiency states
Candidiasis	Vitamin B
Erythema migrans	Folate
Lichen planus	Iron
• Psychogenic	• Diabetes mellitus
Cancerophobia	• Dry mouth
Depression	• Drugs (such as captopril)
Anxiety	• Denture problems
Hypochondriasis	• Parafunctional habits

• Erythema migrans commonly affects the tongue, there are usually no serious connotations, and there is no effective treatment
• Burning mouth syndrome is common, affects mainly the tongue, and antidepressants may be indicated, though organic disease must first be excluded

Orofacial pain

Most orofacial pain is caused by
- Local disease, especially dental, mainly a consequence of caries (see earlier article)
- Psychogenic states
- Neurological disorders (such as trigeminal neuralgia). Similar features are seen in the rare SUNCT syndrome (short lasting, unilateral, neuralgiform headache attacks with conjunctival injection and tearing)
- Vascular disorders (such as migraine). Recent evidence suggests that chronic pain may occasionally be related to thrombosis or hypofibrinolysis causing small areas of jaw ischaemia and necrosis; this has been termed neuralgia-inducing cavitational necrosis
- Referred pain (such as angina).

Causes of orofacial pain

Local diseases
- Teeth and supporting tissues
- Jaws
- Maxillary antrum
- Salivary glands
- Eyes

Psychogenic pain
- Atypical facial pain and other oral symptoms associated with anxiety or depression (such as mandibular pain-dysfunction)
- Burning mouth syndrome

Referred pain
- Angina
- Lesions in neck or chest (including lung cancer)

Neurological disorders
- Trigeminal neuralgia
- Malignant neoplasms
- Multiple sclerosis
- Herpes zoster
- SUNCT syndrome

Vascular disorders
- Migraine
- Migrainous neuralgia
- Temporal arteritis (giant cell arteritis)
- Paroxysmal hemicrania
- Neuralgia-inducing cavitational osteonecrosis

Psychogenic orofacial pain

This is an ill defined entity that includes burning mouth syndrome, atypical facial pain, atypical odontalgia, and the syndrome of oral complaints.

The pain is often of a dull, boring, or burning type of ill defined location. Most patients are women who are middle aged or older. They typically have constant chronic discomfort or pain, rarely use analgesics, sleep undisturbed by pain, have consulted several clinicians, have no objective signs and have negative investigations, and have recent adverse life events such as bereavement or family illness and also multiple psychogenic related complaints.

Management—Attempts at relieving pain by restorative treatment, endodontia, or exodontia are usually unsuccessful. Many patients lack insight and will persist in blaming organic diseases for their pain. Some patients are depressed or hypochondriacal and may respond to fluoxetine or dosulepin hydrochloride. However, many refuse drugs or psychiatric help. Those who will respond invariably do so early in treatment.

Atypical odontalgia presents with pain and hypersensitive teeth typically indistinguishable from pulpitis or periodontitis but without detectable pathology. It is probably a variant of atypical facial pain and should be treated similarly.

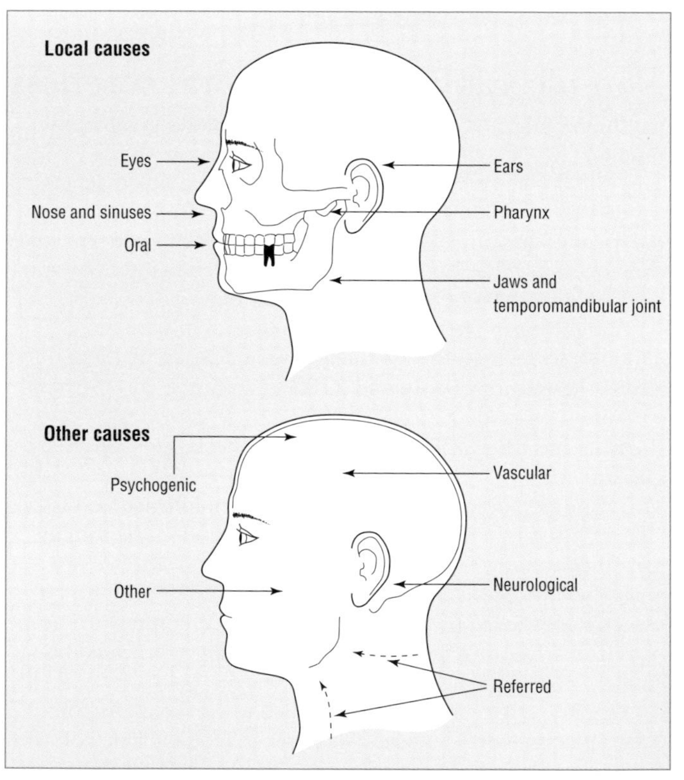

Causes of orofacial pain

Temporomandibular joint pain-dysfunction syndrome (myofascial pain-dysfunction syndrome, facial arthromyalgia)

This common disorder afflicts young women mainly. Symptoms are highly variable but characterised by
- Recurrent clicking in the temporomandibular joint at any point of jaw movement, and there may be crepitus especially with lateral movements
- Periods of limitation of jaw movement, with variable jaw deviation or locking but rarely severe trismus
- Pain in the joint and surrounding muscles, which may be tender to palpation.

Patients with a night time habit of clenching or grinding the teeth (bruxism) may awake with joint pain which abates during the day. In people who clench or grind during working hours the symptoms tend to worsen towards evening and sometimes have a psychogenic basis.

Different aetiological factors that have been implicated include muscle overactivity (such as bruxism and clenching), disruption of the temporomandibular joint, and psychological stress (such as anxiety and stressful life events). Precipitating factors may include wide mouth opening, local trauma, nail biting, and emotional upset. However, there is rarely one specific aetiology, and a combination of factors is often contributory. Occlusal factors do not in general seem to be important.

- **Atypical facial pain and mandibular pain-dysfunction are common forms of orofacial pain**
- **There is typically a poorly localised dull ache**
- **Organic disease must be excluded**
- **Antidepressants may be indicated**

Diagnosis—This is clinical. Radiographic changes are uncommon, and arthrography or magnetic resonance imaging is seldom indicated.

Management—Most patients recover spontaneously, and therefore reassurance and conservative measures are the main management. These include rest, jaw exercises (opening and closing), a soft diet, and analgesics. If these are insufficient, it can be helpful to use plastic splints on the occlusal surfaces (occlusal splints) to reduce joint loading, heat, ultrasound treatment, anxiolytic agents, or antidepressants. A very small minority of patients fail to respond to the above measures and require local corticosteroid or sclerosant therapy, local nerve destruction, or, often as a last resort, joint surgery.

Further reading

- Krause I, Rosen Y, Kaplan I, Milo G, Guedj D, Molad Y, et al. Recurrent aphthous stomatitis in Behcet's disease: clinical features and correlation with systemic disease expression and severity. *J Oral Pathol Med* 1999;28:193-6
- Marbach JJ. Medically unexplained chronic orofacial pain. Temporomandibular pain and dysfunction syndrome, orofacial phantom pain, burning mouth syndrome, and trigeminal neuralgia. *Med Clin North Am* 1999;83:691-710, vi-vii
- Porter SR, Scully C, Pedersen A. Recurrent aphthous stomatitis. *Crit Rev Oral Biol Med* 1998;9:306-21
- Sakane T, Takeno M, Suzuki N, Inaba G. Behcet's disease. *N Engl J Med* 1999;341;1284-91
- Scully C. A review of common mucocutaneous disorders affecting the mouth and lips. *Ann Acad Med Singapore* 1999;28:704-7
- Scully C, Flint S, Porter SR. *Oral diseases.* London: Martin Dunitz, 1996
- Tammiala-Salonen T, Forssell H. Trazodone in burning mouth pain: a placebo-controlled, double-blind study. *J Orofac Pain* 1999;13:83-8
- Van der Waal I. *The burning mouth syndrome.* Copenhagen: Munksgaard, 1990

6 Swellings and red, white, and pigmented lesions

Crispian Scully, Stephen Porter

Swellings

It is not unknown for people to discover and worry about oral lumps, but they usually first notice a lump because it becomes sore. Pathological causes include a range of different lesions, but neoplasms are most important (see earlier article).

Most salivary swellings are caused by mucoceles in minor glands in the lower lip. These are best removed surgically. In the major glands salivary duct obstruction is more common, but sialadenitis, Sjogren's syndrome, and neoplasms are important causes to be excluded. It can be difficult to establish whether a salivary gland is genuinely swollen, especially in obese patients. A useful guide to whether a patient has parotid enlargement is to look for outward deflection of the ear lobe, which is seen in true parotid swelling.

Management—Diagnosis is mainly clinical, but investigations such as serology for autoantibodies or HIV antibodies, liver function tests, and needle or open biopsy may be indicated. Treatment is of the underlying cause.

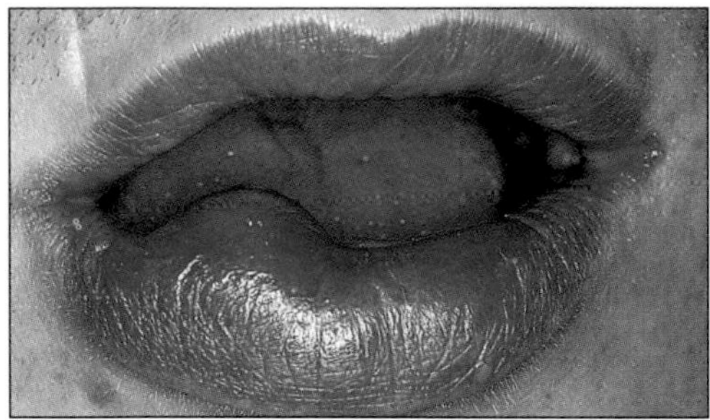

Mucocele in a typical site

Causes of salivary gland swelling

- Inflammatory (mumps, ascending sialadenitis, recurrent juvenile parotitis, HIV sialadenitis, other infections such as tuberculosis, Sjogren's syndrome, sarcoidosis)
- Cystic fibrosis
- Neoplasms
- Duct obstruction
- Sialosis
- Drugs (such as protease inhibitors)
- Deposits (such as amyloid)

Lesions which may present as lumps or swellings in the mouth

Normal
- Pterygoid hamulus
- Parotid papillae
- Lingual papillae
- Unerupted teeth

Developmental
- Haemangioma
- Lymphangioma
- Maxillary and mandibular tori
- Hereditary gingival fibromatosis
- Von Recklinghausen's neurofibromatosis

Inflammatory
- Abscess
- Pyogenic granuloma
- Crohn's disease
- Orofacial granulomatosis
- Sarcoidosis
- Wegener's granulomatosis
- Others

Traumatic
- Epulis
- Fibroepithelial polyp
- Denture granulomas

Cystic
- Eruption cysts
- Developmental cysts
- Cysts of infective origin

Fibro-osseous
- Fibrous dysplasia
- Paget's disease

Hormonal
- Pregnancy epulis or gingivitis
- Oral contraceptive pill gingivitis

Drugs
- Phenytoin
- Cyclosporin
- Calcium channel blockers

Blood dyscrasias
- Leukaemia and lymphoma

Neoplasms
- Benign and malignant

Others
- Angio-oedema
- Amyloidosis

Red oral lesions

Most red oral lesions are inflammatory in nature, but some are potentially malignant, especially erythroplasia.

Erythroplasia (erythroplakia)

Erythroplasia is a rare, isolated, red, velvety lesion that affects patients mainly in their 60s and 70s. It usually involves the floor of the mouth, the ventrum of the tongue, or the soft palate. This is one of the most important oral lesions because 75-90% of lesions prove to be carcinoma or carcinoma in situ or are severely dysplastic. The incidence of malignant change is 17 times higher in erythroplasia than in leucoplakia. Erythroplasia should be excised and sent for histological examination.

• Erythroplasia is an isolated red lesion that typically occurs in elderly people
• It is usually dysplastic or malignant and is best removed

Causes of red lesions

Widespread redness
- Candidiasis
- Iron deficiency
- Avitaminosis B
- Irradiation mucositis
- Lichen planus
- Mucosal atrophy
- Polycythaemia

Localised red patches
- Candidiasis
- Erythroplasia
- Purpura
- Telangiectases
- Angiomas
- Kaposi's sarcoma
- Burns
- Lichen planus
- Lupus erythematosus
- Avitaminosis

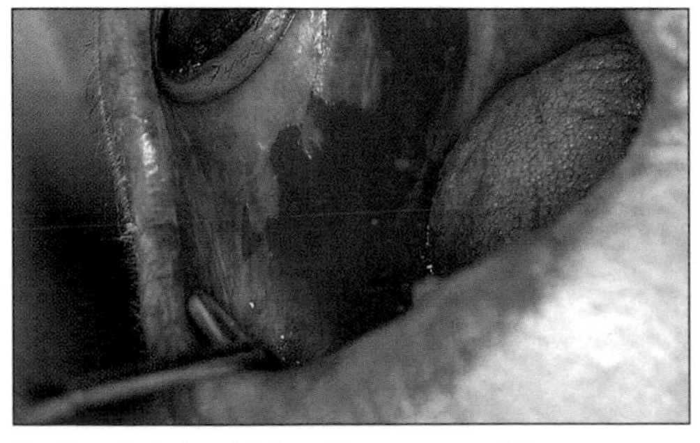

Erythroplasia has high malignant potential

Erythematous candidiasis

Erythematous candidiasis may complicate treatment with corticosteroids or antimicrobials and cause widespread erythema and soreness of the oral mucosa, sometimes with thrush. It may also occasionally be seen in HIV infection, xerostomia, diabetes, and in people who smoke.

Red persistent lesions are especially noticeable on the palate and tongue. Median rhomboid glossitis (central papillary atrophy) is a red depapillated rhomboidal area in the centre of the tongue dorsum, now believed to be associated with candidiasis. Biopsy may show pseudoepitheliomatous hyperplasia, but the condition is not potentially malignant.

Management—Erythematous candidiasis may respond to stopping smoking and antifungal agents (usually fluconazole).

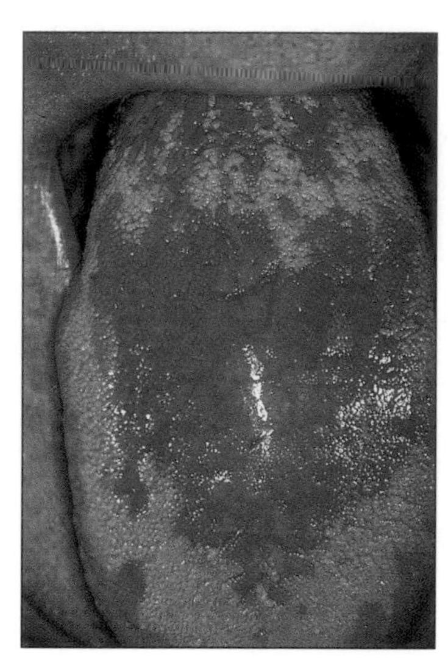

Erythematous candidiasis in patient with HIV infection

Denture induced stomatitis (denture sore mouth)

This is a common form of mild chronic erythematous candidiasis, usually seen after middle age as erythema limited to the area beneath an upper denture. The fitting surface of the denture is infested mainly with *Candida albicans*. Despite its name, this condition is rarely sore, though angular stomatitis may be associated. Patients are usually otherwise healthy.

Factors that predispose to denture induced stomatitis include wearing dentures (especially through the night), poor oral and denture hygiene, xerostomia, and carbohydrate-rich diets. It is not caused by allergy to the denture material.

Management includes

- Eradicating infection by soaking dentures overnight in chlorhexidine or 1% (v/v) hypochlorite solution then using miconazole denture lacquer. Metal dentures should not be soaked in hypochlorite as they may discolour
- Using miconazole gel (5 ml), nystatin pastilles (100 000 units), or amphotericin lozenges (10 mg) in the mouth four times daily for up to one month
- Using systemic fluconazole 50 mg daily for resistant cases
- Adjustment of the dentures.

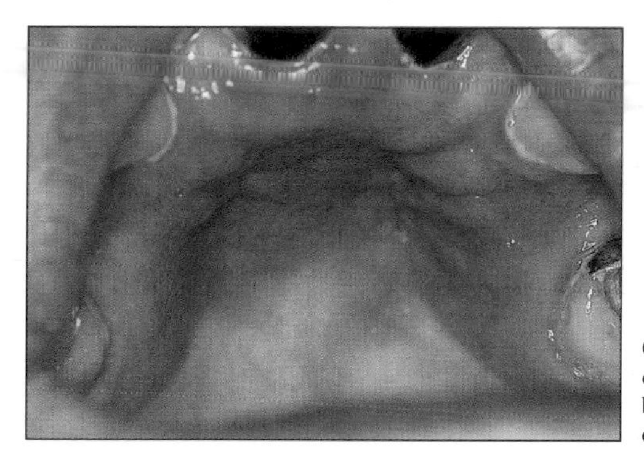

Chronic atrophic candidiasis beneath an upper denture

• Denture stomatitis occurs mainly when *Candida* spp proliferate beneath and infest the denture
• It may be asymptomatic but may be associated with angular stomatitis
• Denture wearing should be minimised and the infection eradicated

Other red lesions

Petechiae are usually caused by trauma or suction but may also be seen in thrombocytopenia, amyloidosis, localised oral purpura, or scurvy. Telangiectasia may be a feature of hereditary haemorrhagic telangiectasia or systemic sclerosis.

White oral lesions

White lesions were formerly called leucoplakia and believed often to be potentially malignant. The term leucoplakia is now restricted to white lesions of unknown cause. Most white lesions are innocuous keratoses caused by cheek biting, friction, or tobacco use, but other conditions must be excluded, usually by biopsy. These include infections (such as candidiasis, syphilis, and hairy leucoplakia), dermatoses (usually lichen planus), and neoplastic disorders (such as leucoplakias and carcinomas). Chronic candidiasis may produce tough, adherent white patches (chronic hyperplastic candidiasis or candidal leucoplakias), which can have a malignant potential and may clinically be indistinguishable from other leucoplakias, though they may be speckled.

Main causes of white oral lesions

- Idiopathic keratosis
- Carcinoma
- Skin grafts
- Physical or chemical
  Friction
  Burns
  Chemicals
  Tobacco
  Snuff
  Sanguinarine
- Infections
  Candidiasis
  Hairy leucoplakia
  Syphilitic keratosis
  Papillomas (some)
- Mucocutaneous disease
  Lichen planus
  Lupus erythematosus
  Inherited lesions (such as white sponge naevus)

Keratosis (leucoplakia)

This is a persistent adherent white patch. Keratoses are most commonly uniformly white plaques (homogenous leucoplakia), prevalent in the buccal mucosae, and are usually of low malignant potential. More serious are non-homogenous keratoses (nodular and, especially, speckled leucoplakias), which consist of white patches or nodules often in a red, commonly eroded, area of mucosa. The presence of severe epithelial dysplasia indicates a considerable risk of malignant development. The overall prevalence of malignant change is

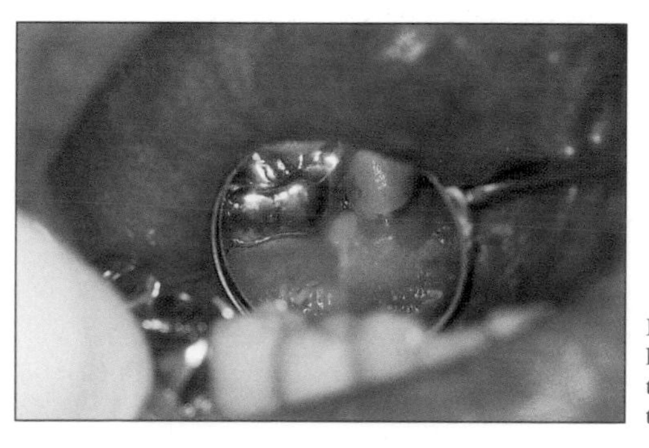

Leucoplakia of lower gingivae—a typical site for this type of lesion

3-33% over 10 years, but a proportion of such malignancies (about 15%) regress spontaneously.

It can be difficult to be certain of the precise diagnosis of a white patch, as even carcinoma can present as a white lesion. Biopsy is indicated, and indurated, red, erosive, or ulcerated areas should be sampled rather than the more obvious whiter hyperkeratinised areas; staining with toluidine blue may help highlight the most appropriate area. An oral brush biopsy may be helpful, but incisional biopsy is needed if carcinoma is strongly suspected.

Management can be difficult, especially in extensive lesions of leucoplakia and those with areas of erythroplasia. Obvious predisposing factors must be reduced or eliminated. Some studies have shown regression of leucoplakia in over half of patients who stopped smoking for a year. Others have shown vitamin A and various retinoids to have beneficial effects, but these are teratogenic and may have other adverse effects such as hyperlipidaemia, and often produce only temporary benefit. Dysplastic lesions should be excised (laser is useful), and patients should then be followed up regularly at intervals of 3-6 months. Unfortunately, excised lesions sometimes recur.

• The aetiology of leucoplakia is unclear
• Less than a third of lesions turn malignant in 10 years
• It is good practice to exclude dysplasia by biopsy
• Leucoplakia is best removed

Lichen planus

Oral lichen planus is common, mainly occurs after middle age, and typically presents as bilateral white lesions (papules, plaques, or reticular areas) in the buccal and lingual mucosae. Lesions may be symptomless. The less common but painful erosive lichen planus typically affects the tongue or buccal mucosae on both sides.

Biopsy is usually necessary to exclude dysplasia, keratosis, lupus erythematosus, chronic ulcerative stomatitis associated with autoantibodies to nuclear proteins (CUSP), and other disorders. Some lichenoid lesions may be drug induced (such as by non-steroidal anti-inflammatory drugs) or occasionally related to factors such as materials used in dental work, hepatitis C infection, or graft versus host disease.

Management—Topical corticosteroids are useful in controlling symptoms. In view of the slight risk (about 1%) of oral carcinoma in non-reticular lichen planus, patients should be regularly reviewed.

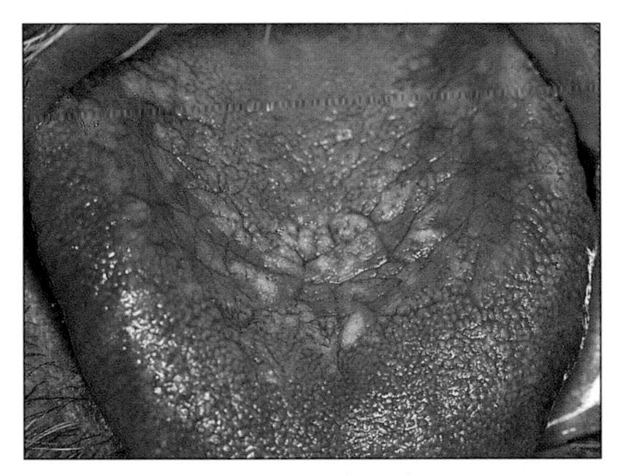

Lichen planus of dorsum of tongue

• Lichen planus is common
• There is no single cause, but it is often idiopathic and may be related to drug use or dental materials.
• Diagnosis from leucoplakia and lupus erythematosus can be difficult
• It is often treated with topical corticosteroids

Candidiasis (candidosis, moniliasis, thrush)

Oral carriage of *Candida albicans* is more common in people who smoke and those who are ill. *C albicans* is the most common cause of candidiasis, which can arise in patients after recent use of antibiotics or corticosteroids, immunosuppressive drugs, cytotoxic chemotherapy, or irradiation; in those with xerostomia, immunodeficiencies such as leukaemia or AIDS, malnutrition, or diabetes; and in neonates, who have little immunity to *Candida* spp. The soft, creamy patches of thrush can be wiped off the mucosa, leaving erythema.

Management—Avoid smoking, treat predisposing causes (such as xerostomia), and improve oral hygiene. Chlorhexidine has some anti-candidal activity, and antifungal drugs can be used, the choice depending on the severity and extent of disease, medical contraindications, and other complications of an immunocompromising condition.

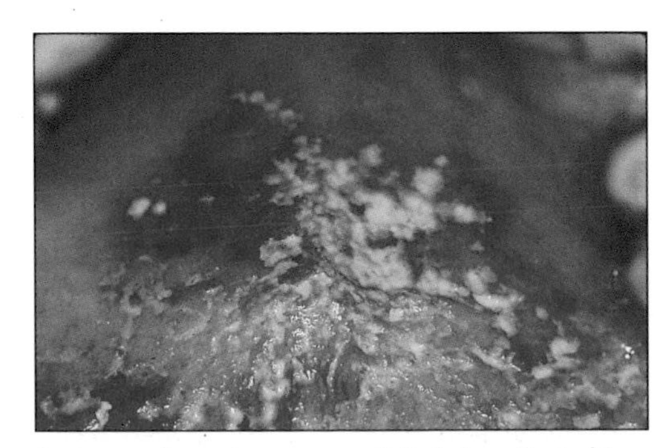

Acute pseudomembranous candidiasis in patient with drug induced immunosuppression

• Candidiasis may be seen in healthy neonates
• It otherwise indicates local immunosuppressive treatment, xerostomia, or an immune defect

Hairy leucoplakia

This is an asymptomatic white lesion not removable by wiping that is typically seen on the lateral margins of the tongue in immunocompromised patients, usually those with HIV infection or AIDS. It is associated with Epstein-Barr virus and has no known malignant potential, but it is a predictor of poor prognosis and, in HIV infection, is an AIDS-defining condition.

Treatment is usually not required, but it resolves with aciclovir or anti-retroviral agents.

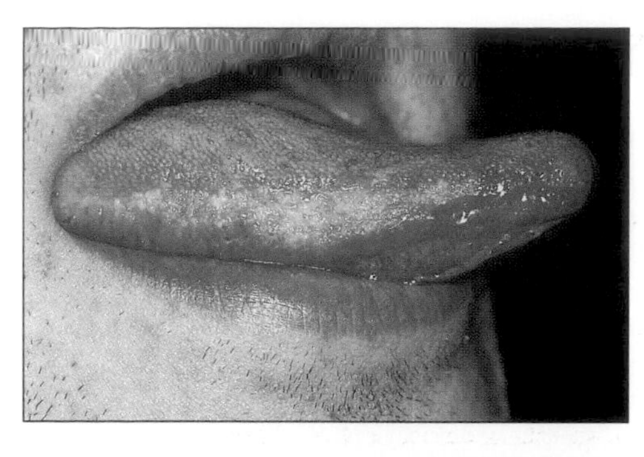

Hairy leucoplakia on lateral margin of tongue of patient with AIDS

Pigmented oral lesions

Furred, brown, and black hairy tongue

The tongue in healthy children is seldom furred, but healthy adults sometimes have a coating of epithelial, food, and microbial debris, particularly if they are edentulous, have a soft non-abrasive diet, have poor oral hygiene, smoke, are fasting or ill, or are using antimicrobials or chlorhexidine. Black hairy tongue is an extreme example that affects mainly the posterior dorsum of tongue. The filiform papillae are long and stained by accumulated debris.

Management—The condition is improved by increasing oral hygiene, brushing the tongue, using a tongue scraper, increasing dietary fruit and roughage (pineapple may help), and using sodium bicarbonate mouthwashes.

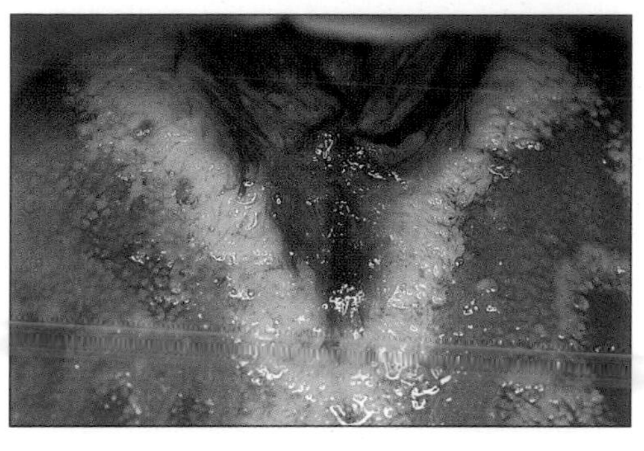

Black hairy tongue in patient who, by chance, also has erythema migrans (see previous article)

Localised hyperpigmented lesions

Haemangiomas, purpura, and Kaposi's sarcoma give rise to localised red and purple lesions. Brown or black lesions are usually amalgam tattoos or naevi, but melanomas must be excluded.

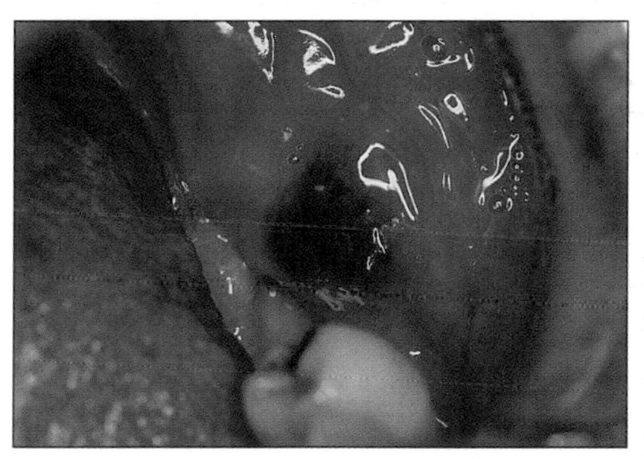

Haemangioma of left buccal mucosa. Unlike Kaposi's sarcoma, this lesion blanches on pressure

Generalised mucosal hyperpigmentation

This is usually racial in origin or caused by smoking or betel use and only occasionally has a systemic cause such as drugs, Addison's disease, or ectopic production of adrenocorticotrophic hormone (such as by bronchogenic carcinoma).

- **Hyperpigmentation in the buccal cavity may be due to racial origin or caused by dental amalgam, drugs, using tobacco or betel, naevi, or, rarely, melanoma**
- **Brown tongue is usually caused by poor diet or oral hygiene**

Causes of brown or black pigmented mucosal lesions

- Ephelis (freckle)
- Racial
- Naevus
- Malignant melanoma
- Kaposi's sarcoma
- Peutz-Jegher's syndrome
- Amalgam or graphite tattoo
- Drugs (such as phenothiazines, zidovudine, minocycline)
- Smoking
- Heavy metals
- Addison's disease (and related disorders)
- Other rare causes

Further reading

- Lee LA, Walsh P, Prater CA, Su LJ, Marchbank A, Egbert TB, et al. Characterization of an autoantigen associated with chronic ulcerative stomatitis: the CUSP autoantigen is a member of the p53 family. *J Invest Dermatol* 1999;113:146-51
- Mashberg A. Early diagnosis of asymptomatic oral and oropharyngeal squamous cancers. *CA Cancer J Clin* 1995;45:328-51
- Schoelch ML, Sekandari N, Regezi JA, Silverman S. Laser management of oral leukoplakias: a follow-up study of 70 patients. *Laryngoscope* 1999;109:949-53
- Sciubba JJ. Improving detection of precancerous and cancerous oral lesions: computer-assisted analysis of the oral brush biopsy. *J Am Dent Assoc* 1999;130:1445-57
- Scully C, Beyli M, Feirrero M, Ficarra G, Gill Y, Griffiths M, et al. Update on oral lichen planus: aetiopathogenesis and management. *Crit Rev Oral Biol Med* 1998;9:86-122
- Scully C, Cawson RA. Potentially malignant oral lesions. *J Epidemiol Biostatistics* 1996;1:3-12
- Scully C, Flint S, Porter SR. *Oral diseases.* London: Martin Dunitz, 1996
- Triantos D, Porter SR, Scully C, Teo CG. Oral hairy leukoplakia; clinicopathological features, pathogenesis, diagnosis and clinical significance. *Clin Infect Dis* 1997;25:1392-6

7 Improving occlusion and orofacial aesthetics: orthodontics

Susan Cunningham, Elisabeth Horrocks, Nigel Hunt, Steven Jones, Howard Moseley, Joseph Noar, Crispian Scully

Malocclusion is the abnormal positioning of the teeth or jaws. It is a variation of growth and development and can affect a person's bite (occlusion), ability to clean teeth properly, gingival health, jaw growth, speech development, and appearance.

The shape and size of the face, jaws, and teeth are mainly inherited, but environmental factors can also have an impact. Factors as diverse as skeletal muscle pathology[1] and sucking a digit (thumb or finger) can substantially influence the growth of the face and dentition.

Treatment of disorders such as crowded or protruding teeth may improve both aesthetics and oral function. In addition, prominent teeth can be damaged easily during childhood. The dental specialty most concerned with problems of facial growth, development of occlusion, and the prevention and correction of associated anomalies is orthodontics. The improvement of occlusion and aesthetics using restorative dental techniques is discussed in the next article.

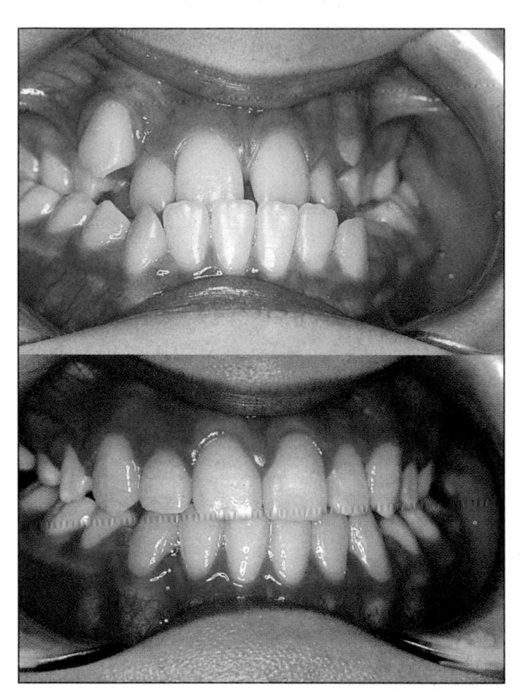

Patient with crowded teeth and malocclusion (top) and after orthodontic treatment (bottom)

Orthodontic care

The demand for orthodontic treatment is increasing to such an extent that an objective index of orthodontic treatment need (IOTN) has been established to ensure that resources are directed to patients with the greatest clinical need and who are likely to benefit most.[2 3]

Apart from a thorough history and examination, photographs of the face and teeth and models of the teeth are used to provide a record and facilitate treatment planning. Several types of radiograph may also be needed. Most commonly used are panoramic radiographs, which show all the upper and lower teeth in biting position as well as any teeth still developing within the jaws, and a lateral cephalometric radiograph, which shows the relation of the teeth and jaws to the face and base of the skull.

Prevention or treatment of malocclusion may help
- **Aesthetic appearance**
- **Occlusion**
- **Oral health**
- **Reduce dental trauma**

Treatment

Tooth extraction

Carefully controlled removal of selected primary teeth may be prescribed to facilitate the eruption of the permanent teeth into their correct position. Orthodontic treatment may also require healthy permanent teeth to be extracted when there is dento-alveolar disproportion—that is, a discrepancy in the size of the jaw in relation to the teeth present. Some malocclusions cannot be treated successfully without removing permanent teeth, though tooth removal is contraindicated in other situations. Typically, premolars are selected for extraction since this maintains aesthetics, but other teeth may be extracted if they are heavily filled, decayed, or have poor long term prognosis. Only very rarely are anterior teeth extracted for orthodontic reasons.

Tooth movement

Treatment involves moving the teeth through the supporting alveolar bone to the desired position. This must be carried out slowly and carefully to avoid pain or damage to the teeth. It is done by means of fixed or removable appliances (braces) that gently move the teeth and supporting alveolar bone until they

- **The index of orthodontic treatment need is frequently used to determine clinical need and potential benefit**
- **Space in the dental arch is gained by tooth movement or extraction**
- **Teeth are generally moved by wires and springs on removable or fixed appliances**
- **Treatment typically takes 18-30 months**
- **Early treatment is often simpler and more effective than later treatment**
- **Timing of referral in children is important**
- **Screening for malocclusion by general dental practitioners is recommended at 9-10 years of age**

are in the desired position. The braces consist of brackets, made of metal, ceramics, or plastic, and an archwire that connects them. The teeth are moved by adjusting the pressures on them via the archwire. Springs or elastic bands may be used to help. The appliances are tightened periodically, and some discomfort is then felt for a few hours. It should be noted that placement and removal of orthodontic bands can cause a transient bacteraemia, and in cases with a risk of infective endocarditis appropriate antibiotic cover should be administered.[4,5]

The length of time required to move teeth to the desired location varies considerably. The average for children is 18-30 months, but it is generally longer for adults. The time required depends on the malocclusion complexity, amount of space available, distance the teeth must move, cooperation of the patient, bone density, and age of the patient.

When the desired occlusion has been achieved and the braces removed, a retainer is used, typically for 6-12 months, to prevent the teeth reverting towards their original positions. In some cases, retention may be needed long term.

Other types of brace include functional appliances which are orthopaedic devices designed to modify jaw growth, particularly in patients with a recessive lower jaw. In some situations additional components, such as extraoral appliances, may be worn to complement fixed or removable appliances, and these are generally worn only during the evening and night.

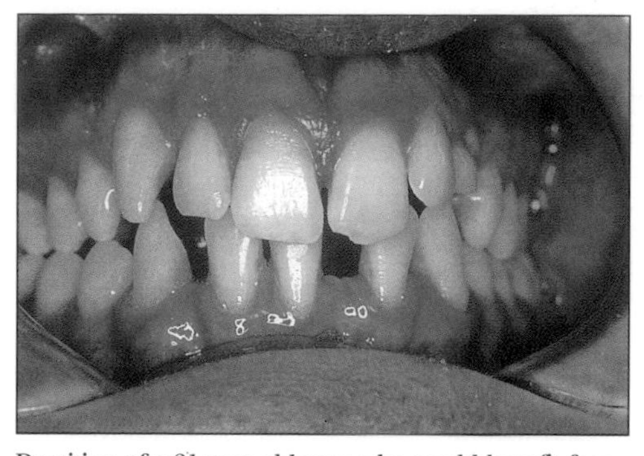

Dentition of a 21 year old man who would benefit from orthodontic treatment to relocate spaces in lower jaw before bridges are placed to correct aesthetic appearance

Orthodontics in children and adolescents

Most orthodontic treatment is carried out during childhood since the teeth can then most readily be moved. Some problems are treated most effectively when the child is actively growing, and, for this reason, the timing of referral is critical. This particularly applies to children with very prominent upper teeth and a small lower jaw. Failure to treat at the appropriate age may mean that orthodontic correction of the problem is not feasible and that the patient will require orthognathic surgery at a later stage. All children should be screened at about 9-10 years of age by their dental practitioner, and appropriate referral for a specialist opinion instigated where necessary.

Orthodontics in adults

Orthodontics is increasingly used in adults. This may involve orthodontics alone or orthodontics together with intervention from another dental discipline. Thus, orthodontic care may be required when teeth need to be moved to allow ideal restorations (such as crowns or bridges) to be placed.

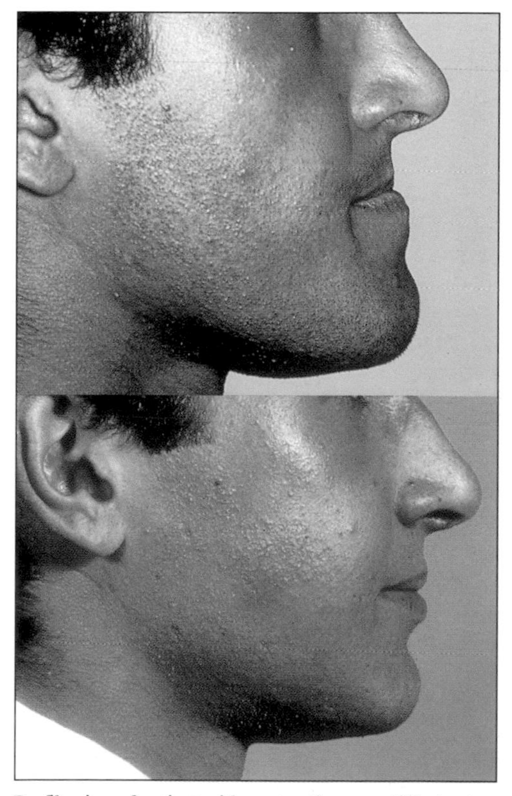

Profile view of patient with protruding mandible (top) and after orthognathic treatment (bottom)

Orthognathic surgery

When there is a severe skeletal discrepancy or there is no growth allowing orthopaedic correction, orthodontics alone will not solve the problem. Patients who present with severe dentofacial problems (such as an extremely recessive or protruding mandible or facial asymmetries) may require a combination of fixed braces to place the teeth in an ideal position followed by maxillofacial surgery to reposition the jaws in the correct relationship (orthognathic treatment). This form of treatment is undertaken when growth is complete and can produce marked improvements in facial and dental appearance and in oral function. These improvements often lead to improvements in patients' self confidence, their ability to interact socially, and how they are perceived by others.[6]

Distraction osteogenesis, the forcible lengthening of bone, is being developed for patients with severe dentofacial problems, including adults and some children with syndromes manifesting severe deformities (such as the midfacial deformity typical of Crouzon syndrome).

- **Severe malocclusions may be disfiguring and not correctable by orthodontics alone**
- **A combination of orthodontics and orthognathic surgery may be indicated**
- **Some malocclusions may be amenable to distraction osteogenesis**

Cleft lip and palate and facial syndromes

Cleft lip and palate

Cleft lip and palate is the most common congenital deformity in the craniofacial region, with an incidence of about 1 in 700 live births. The presentation may range from a bifid uvula, often associated with a submucous cleft, to a complete bilateral cleft of the lip and palate. Submucous clefts are often not recognised early as there is apparently an intact soft palate, but the muscle alignment is abnormal and may give rise to poor speech development.

An orthodontist should attend a baby with cleft lip or palate as soon as possible after birth in order to decide whether to construct a feeding plate and to advise the parents on future management. The child will continue to be seen regularly by the orthodontist and will require intervention at several stages during development as well as careful dental care.

The orthodontist will monitor facial growth and development of the dentition. Active treatment is required before bone grafting of the alveolar palatal defect at about 10 years of age. This timing is dictated by the stage of dental development, when the canine tooth will erupt through the newly placed bone graft. When the permanent teeth have erupted then comprehensive orthodontic treatment is often indicated. There may be extra or missing teeth or teeth with poor prognosis in the site of the cleft. The orthodontist must take all these factors into account when planning definitive treatment, which may involve dental extractions and the use of fixed appliances.

Patients with clefts of the lip and palate often present with facial growth problems, with the maxilla being recessive relative to the mandible, and these patients may well require some form of orthognathic surgery when growth has ceased. As with all stages of treatment, if orthognathic surgery is required this should be planned carefully by the orthodontist, maxillofacial surgeon, otorhinolaryngologist, plastic surgeon, restorative dentist, and speech therapist for optimal results.

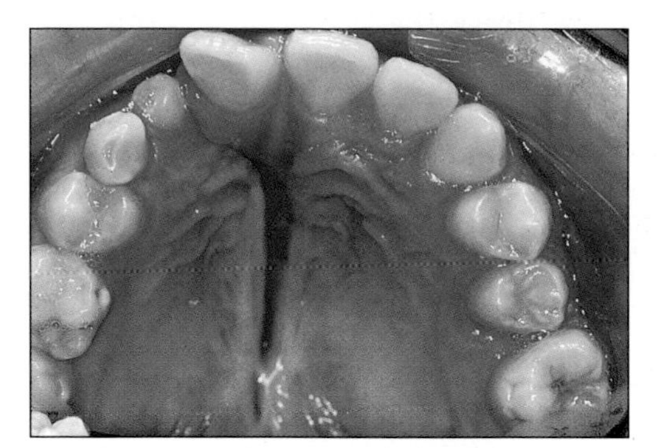

Palatal view of patient with cleft lip and palate

• Management of cleft lip and palate involves a team approach with orthodontists and surgeons in key roles
• Crucial treatment times for a patient with cleft palate are before bone grafting (around 10 years) and when the permanent teeth have erupted

Facial syndromes

Some syndromes affecting the craniofacial region are relatively minor (such as cleidocranial dysplasia), but others are much more severe (such as first arch syndrome, Crouzon syndrome, and Apert syndrome). Many require orthodontic care, conducted in major regional craniofacial centres. Orthodontists also play a role in diagnosing systemic conditions that affect facial growth or development of the dentition, such as acromegaly or Marfan's syndrome. These may require orthodontic or surgical intervention to correct the associated problems.

1 Hunt NP. Muscle function and the control of facial form. In: Harris M, Edgar M, Meghji S, eds. *Clinical oral science.* Oxford: Wright, 1998: 120-33.
2 Brook PH, Shaw WC. The development of an index of orthodontic treatment priority. *Eur J Orthod* 1989;11:309-20.
3 Otuyemi OD, Jones SP. Methods of assessing and grading malocclusion: A review. *Aust Orthod J* 1995;14:21-7.
4 Erverdi N, Kadir T, Ozkan H, Acar A. Investigation of bacteremia after orthodontic banding. *Am J Orthod Dentofacial Orthop* 1999;116:687-90.
5 Khurana M, Martin MV. Orthodontics and infective endocarditis. *Br J Orthod* 1999;26:295-8.
6 Cunningham SJ, Hunt NP, Feinmann C. Psychological aspects of orthognathic surgery—A review of the literature. *Int J Adult Orthod Orthognath Surg* 1995;10:159-72.

8 Improving occlusion and orofacial aesthetics: tooth repair and replacement

Ken Hemmings, Brigitte Griffiths, John Hobkirk, Crispian Scully

There have been tremendous advances in restorative dentistry, particularly with the development of adhesive materials to replace lost tooth structure and jaw implants on which to place prostheses securely.

Repair of teeth

Individuals vary in tooth shade and shape, and teeth yellow with age. Teeth are damaged by caries, wear, failed restorations, trauma, and congenital and developmental defects. Patients usually demand treatment for pain, when appearance is compromised, or when there are occlusal problems (see previous article)

Restorative dental care is indicated to treat pain, poor aesthetic appearance, and poor occlusal function

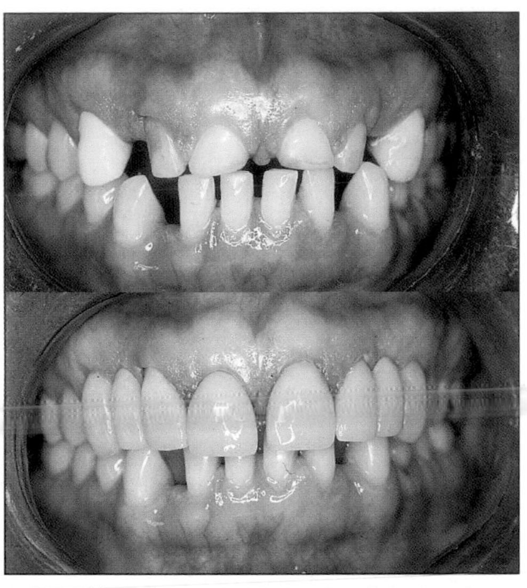

Patient with badly worn and spaced teeth (top) and appearance after restoration (bottom)

Restorations

Most older adults have had restorations (fillings), but, with the benefits of health education and fluoride, many younger people have unrestored teeth.

Most restorations are placed to treat caries. The decay is removed mechanically, the cavity shaped to retain the filling, and material is packed into the cavity and then sets hard. Even high quality restorations have a finite life span. If the pulp is diseased, root canal treatment is necessary, which involves removing the pulp and cleansing and filling the chamber.

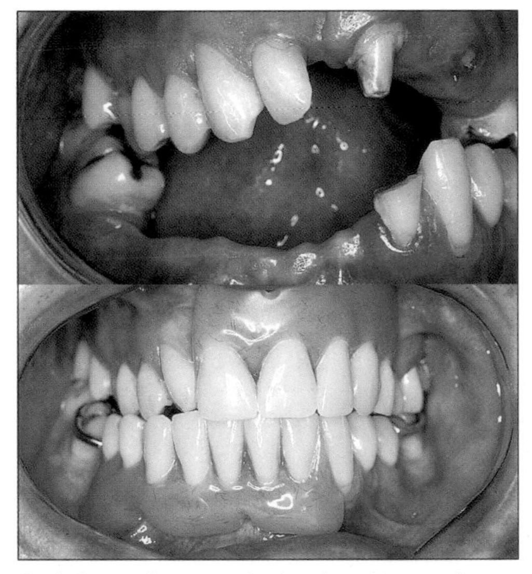

Tooth damage by trauma (top) and appearance after restoration (bottom)

Amalgam

Amalgam contains silver, copper, tin, and zinc mixed with mercury, and sets within a few minutes. Exposure to mercury vapour is hazardous. Mercury is neurotoxic, and even in people with low level chronic exposure, subtle preclinical effects on symptoms, mood, motor function, and cognition have been identified. Pregnant dental staff have special concerns related to any daily occupational exposure to mercury (or nitrous oxide).

However, any risk to patients from dental amalgams is less clear. Twenty two million amalgams are placed annually in the United Kingdom, with no reliable evidence of associations with systemic disease, although a few patients have allergies or lichenoid oral reactions. Austria, Germany, and Sweden have restricted amalgam use, but removal of amalgam on health grounds diagnosed by a dentist is unethical. There is no reliable evidence for implicating amalgam in Alzheimer's disease, autoimmune diseases, birth defects, digestive disturbances, multiple sclerosis, or Parkinson's disease.

Amalgam has physical properties superior to tooth coloured materials, the only reasonable alternatives. It is the most cost effective restorative material, with an average life span of about five years, although some fillings last 20 years or more. Amalgam has been used for over 170 years. Nevertheless, because of the health concerns the UK Department of Health has recently advised that amalgams should not be placed in pregnant women. After assessment of the potential risks of undergoing dental treatment during pregnancy, it can be stated that necessary treatment should not be withheld. Dental

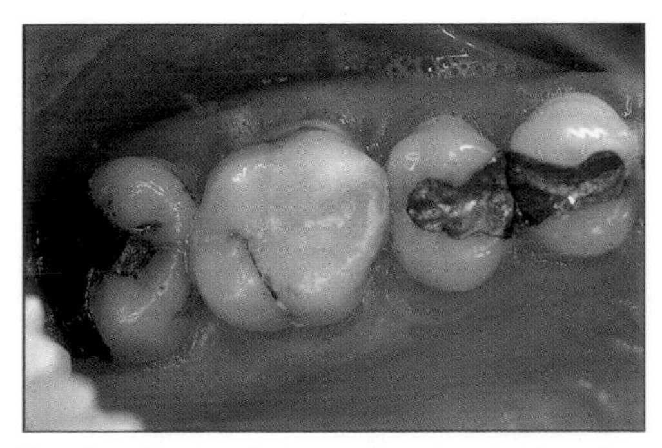

Dental amalgams and a composite restoration in molars to treat caries

treatments are best performed in the second trimester for the benefit of the fetus and optimal comfort of the pregnant woman.

Tooth coloured materials
Tooth coloured materials or "white fillings" are usually either composite resins that adhere to the tooth or glass ionomer cements. They can contain chemicals such as acrylate, peroxides, bisphenol, formaldehyde, hexane, hydroquinone, phenol, polyurethane, silane, toluene, and xylene, some of which have been suspected of toxicity. However, apart from occasional allergic reactions, there is little evidence of adverse effects arising from the placement of tooth coloured fillings. Concerns about an oestrogenic effect, for example, have not been substantiated. These restorations have aesthetic appeal. The disadvantage is they cannot withstand heavy biting forces.

Dental amalgam has been used for more than a century
• Amalgam is stronger and longer lasting than tooth coloured restorations but is less aesthetically pleasing
• There is no reliable evidence of systemic health risk to those with amalgam restorations, but it is recommended that they are not placed or removed in pregnant women

Bleaching
Extrinsic tooth stains can be reduced by scaling and polishing. Intrinsic staining is difficult to remove. The enamel surface can be removed by rotary instruments, microabrasion sandblasting with aluminum oxide, or polishing with pumice in acid. Bleaching with carbamide peroxide gel in a gum shield is effective for mild discolourations.

Tetracycline staining is now much reduced after the avoidance of its use in pregnant and lactating women and children under 12 years old.

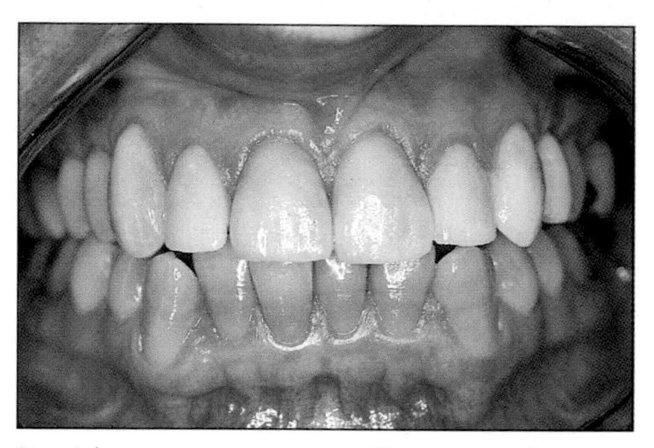

Porcelain veneers to treat tetracycline staining of upper teeth (appearance of lower teeth was deemed acceptable)

Veneers
Porcelain or composite veneers stuck on the tooth surface can improve their shape and shade for up to 10 years. Minimal preparation is required.

Crowns
Crowns are indicated when little tooth material remains. Crowns generally cover all or much of the tooth crown and are the same size and shape as the original tooth, unless that was malformed or misaligned. Crowns are cemented on the teeth, are not removable by the patient, and can withstand chewing. Full gold or non-precious metal alloy crowns are often prescribed for posterior teeth.

Gold crowns, made from gold alloyed with platinum, palladium, copper, silver, and zinc, last from 10 to 20 years. Lichenoid reactions to them occasionally occur.

Non-precious metal crowns (mainly nickel) are stronger and cheaper. Beryllium is often present, giving rise to concern about toxicity to dental laboratory technicians.

All-porcelain crowns give a better aesthetic appearance, but more tooth preparation is required.

Most crowns have porcelain fused to a metal substructure to combine aesthetics with strength.

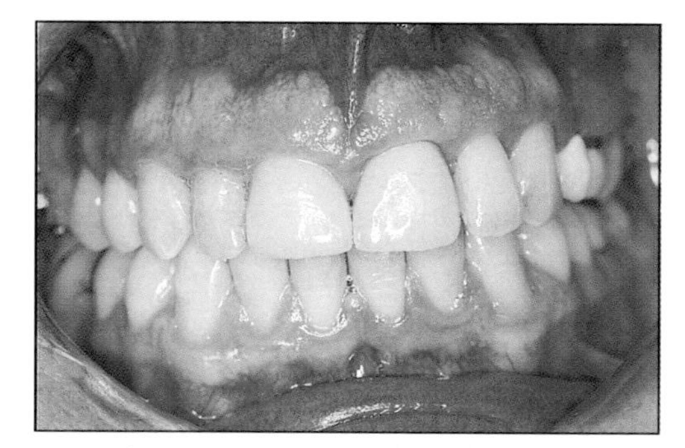

Conventional crown on maxillary left central incisor

Inlays and onlays
These are laboratory made and expensive. They fit a tooth to replace lost tooth material.

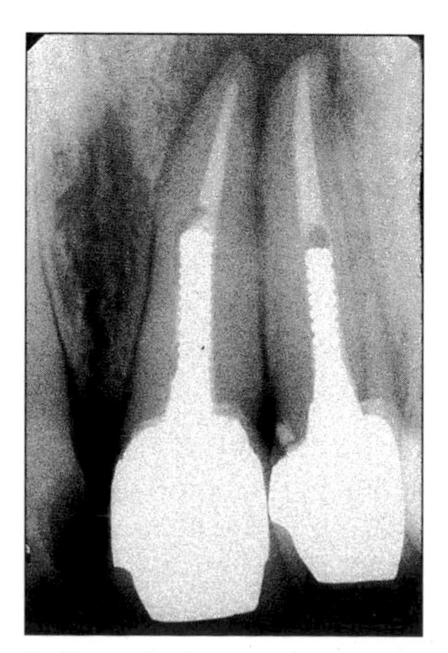

Radiograph of post crowns showing endodontic filling and retaining post

Aesthetic appearance can be improved mainly by
- **Tooth cleaning**
- **Bleaching**
- **Tooth coloured restorations**
- **Veneers**
- **Crowns**

Replacement of teeth

In 1988, 52% of people aged 65-74 years in Britain lacked natural teeth, reflecting the high levels of dental disease in the past. By the year 2008, this percentage is expected to have dropped to about 25%. People lose teeth or have tooth spaces for various reasons, including caries, periodontitis, failed dentistry, trauma, and hypodontia. In general, most people desire replacement of anterior teeth so that they have a reasonable smile. Posterior teeth may need to be replaced to restore occlusion.

All teeth can be replaced with removable partial or complete dentures. Bridgework or fixed tooth replacement is possible when sufficient teeth of good quality remain that can be used as supports for false teeth. Dental implants can replace teeth independently of remaining natural teeth and can replace single teeth as well as complete dental arches.

In general, young patients with relatively unrestored teeth have all options for tooth replacement open to them. Tooth replacement is much more difficult if many teeth are missing or they have been heavily restored.

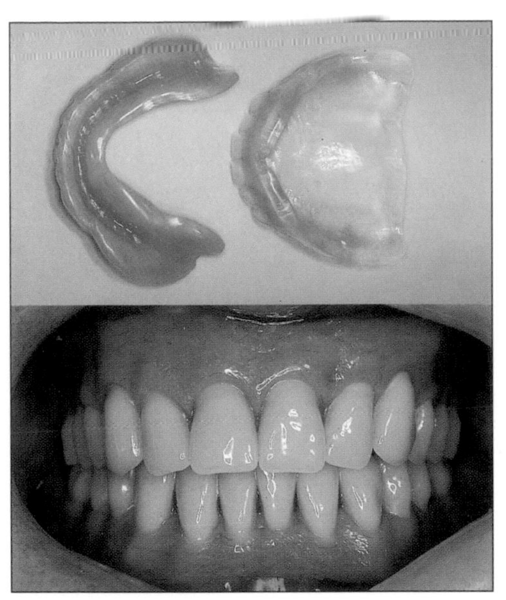

Complete lower and upper dentures (top) and their appearance in situ (bottom)

Missing teeth can be replaced with
- **Removable dentures (placed on mucosa, teeth, roots, or implants)**
- **Non-removable bridges fixed to teeth**
- **Implants in jaw, carrying a denture, crown, or bridge**

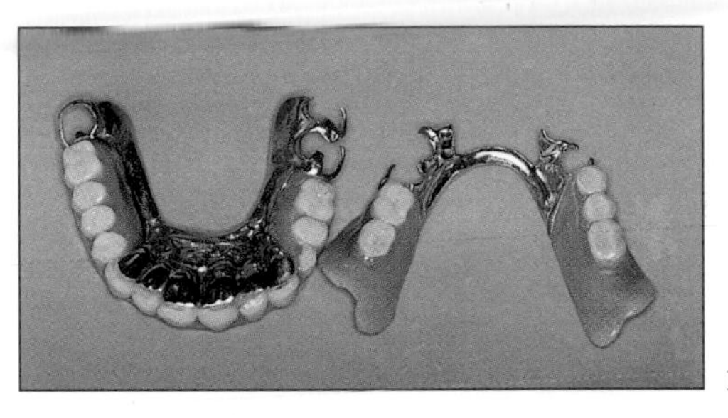

Partial dentures

Dentures

Dentures are removable by the patient and are the most cost effective way of replacing teeth. Dentures are often constructed from plastic (acrylic resin) but may also have cobalt, chromium, or gold components. The cost depends on the complexity of design and materials used. The incidence of allergic responses is extremely low. Maintenance of oral hygiene is fundamental to the success of the treatment.

Complete dentures are retained by adhesion via saliva to the mucosa and the adaptive response of the oral musculature. Most patients have few problems wearing complete upper dentures. The most common complaints are looseness and pain related to a lower denture. Denture problems may increase as the alveolar bone naturally resorbs after tooth extraction or when there is xerostomia or impaired neuromuscular control.

Partial dentures replace teeth in patients who are partially dentate. Metal alloy clasps and rests aid retention and support.

Onlays (overlays, overdentures)—When the dentition is severely worn or only a few teeth remain, dentures may be constructed over the remnants. The advantages in retaining such teeth or roots are that the alveolar bone and proprioception of the roots are maintained and the stability and retention of the denture are improved.

Overdenture (top) supported by metal studs inserted into natural tooth roots (bottom)

Obturators—Palatal defects may be congenital, as in cleft palate, or acquired after tumour excision. Oral function (speech, drinking, and eating) may be severely compromised since air, food, and fluids pass between the mouth and the nose. Dentures incorporating a bung or obturator component provide a seal between the oral and nasal cavities and thus improve function.

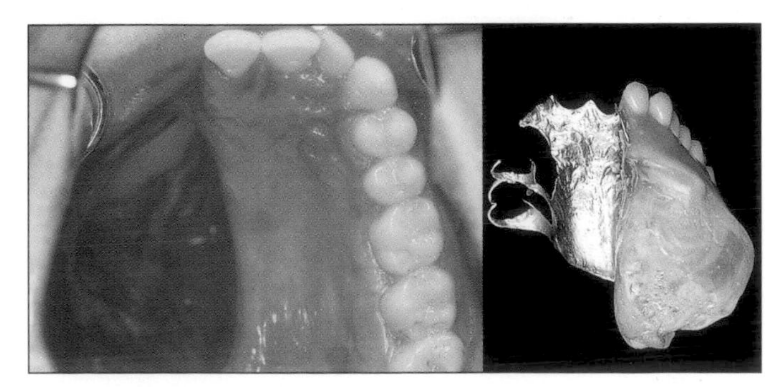

Patient with palatal defect (left) and obturator made to separate oral and nasal cavities (right)

Bridgework

Bridgework involves the preparation of supporting teeth known as abutments. The false tooth or pontic is attached to a crown known as a retainer, and the prosthesis is cemented on to the abutment. The average lifespan for such bridgework is 10 years.

Resin bonded bridgework is secured to the teeth with adhesive composite resin materials. It is indicated when the teeth are relatively unrestored. The main advantage is that little or no tooth preparation is required, and it is particularly suitable for young patients with missing teeth. However, not all teeth can be replaced in this way. The average lifespan is between 5 and 10 years.

Dental implants

Implants provide replacement of missing natural teeth with artificial analogues. Probably the most important development in dentistry, implants can be used singly, to support a crown, or in groups to stabilise dentures or bridges.

A titanium precision screw is surgically inserted into the alveolus where it anchors (a process called osseointegration). After three to six months, an intraoral component or abutment is added to support a prosthesis. These implants have success rates for individual implants of >95% in the lower jaw and >90% in the upper jaw over 10 years. Treatment, however, requires considerable skills and appropriate case selection, planning, clinical procedures, and maintenance.

There are few absolute systemic contraindications to implants. Failure rates increase with diabetes, chemotherapy, tobacco smoking, ectodermal dysplasia, and erosive lichen planus. Implant treatment is expensive, in time and materials, and any contraindication to surgery precludes implants.

Dental implants
- **Are placed surgically in the alveolus**
- **Carry a denture, crown, or bridge**
- **Result in a very stable retentive prosthesis**
- **Have a high success rate (>90% last at least 10 years)**

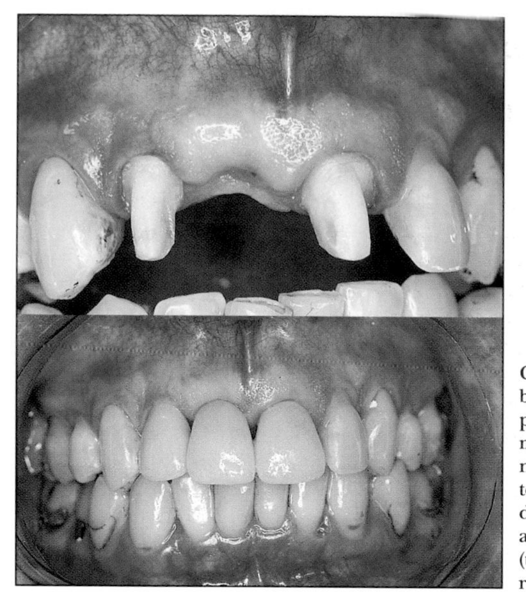

Conventional bridgework in patient with missing incisor: neighbouring teeth are ground down to take artificial crowns (top) and final result (bottom)

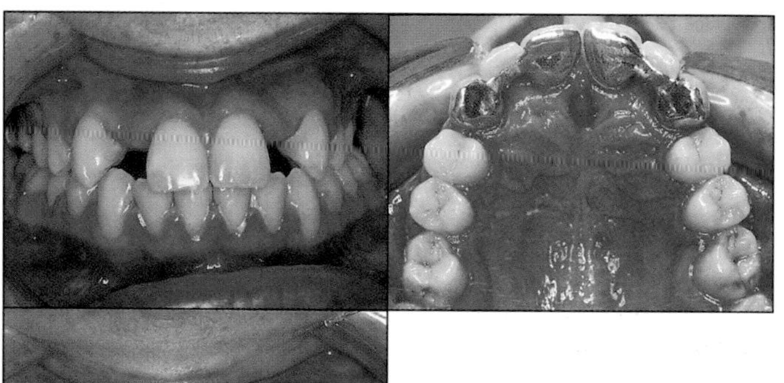

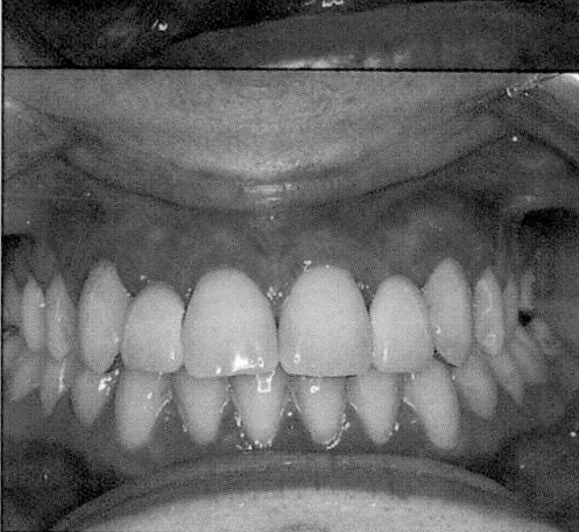

Resin bonded bridgework in patient with hypodontia (top left): with minimal tooth preparation, the metal substructure is glued to the intact teeth (top right) and final result (left)

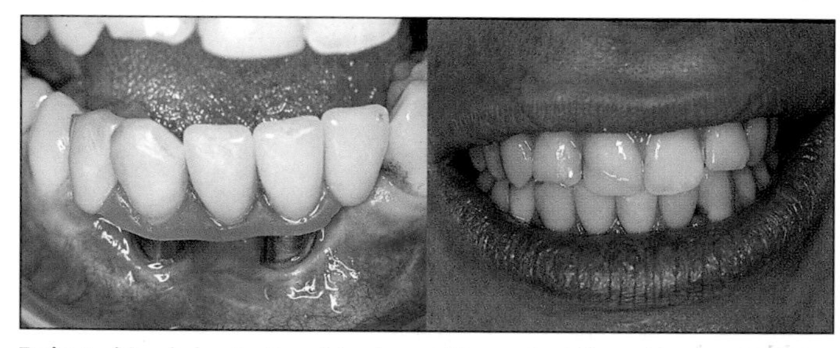

Patient with missing teeth and jaw bone after road traffic accident: temporary appliance on dental implants (left) and definitive prosthesis in place (right)

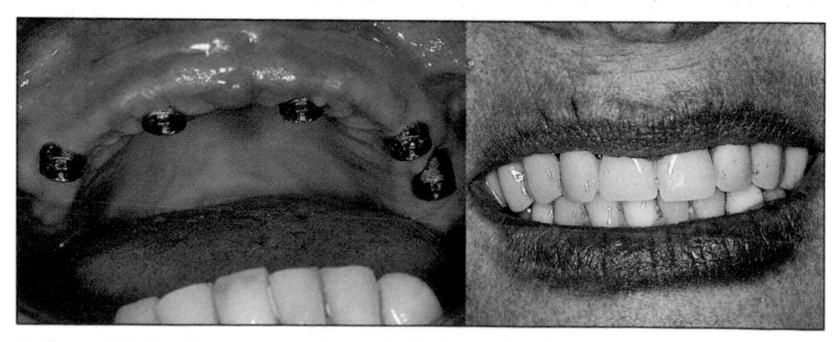

Patient with implants inserted surgically into alveolar bone of edentulous maxilla (left) to stabilise fixed bridge (right)

Further reading

- Albrektsson T, Sennerby L. State of the art in oral implants. *J Clin Periodontol* 1991;18:474-81
- Barclay CW, Walmsley AD. *Fixed and removable prosthodontics.* Edinburgh: Churchill Livingstone, 1998
- Echeverria D, Aposhian HV, Woods JS, Heyer NJ, Aposhian MM, Bittner AC Jr, et al. Neurobehavioral effects from exposure to dental amalgam Hg(o): new distinctions between recent exposure and Hg body burden. *FASEB J* 1998;12:971-80
- Eley BM. The future of dental amalgam: a review of the literature. Part 6: Possible harmful effects of mercury from dental amalgam. *Br Dent J* 1997;182:455-9
- Mount GJ, Hume WR. *Preservation and restoration of tooth structure.* London: Mosby, 1998
- Schmalz G. The biocompatibility of non-amalgam dental filling materials. *Eur J Oral Sci* 1998;106:696-706
- Sheldon T, Treasure E. Dental restoration: what type of filling? *Effective Health Care* 1999;5(2):1-12
- Wasylko L, Matsui D, Dykxhoorn SM, Rieder MJ, Weinberg S. A review of common dental treatments during pregnancy: implications for patients and dental personnel. *J Can Dent Assoc* 1998;64:434-9

9 Oral health care for patients with special needs

Roger Davies, Raman Bedi, Crispian Scully

People with special needs are those whose dental care is complicated by a physical, mental, or social disability. They have tended to receive less oral health care, or of lower quality, than the general population, yet they may have oral problems that can affect systemic health. Improving oral health for people with special needs is possible mainly through community based dental care systems. Education of patients and parents or carers with regard to prevention and treatment of oral disease must be planned from an early stage. This will minimise disease and operative intervention since extractions and surgical procedures in particular often produce major problems. Dental healthcare workers also often need to be educated about this subject.

In this context various conditions can lead to people needing special care, not least patients with dental phobias. Many of these patients can be treated with behavioural modification techniques, though a minority will require sedation or general anaesthesia.

This article concentrates on those who are medically compromised, mentally challenged, mentally ill, or socially excluded.

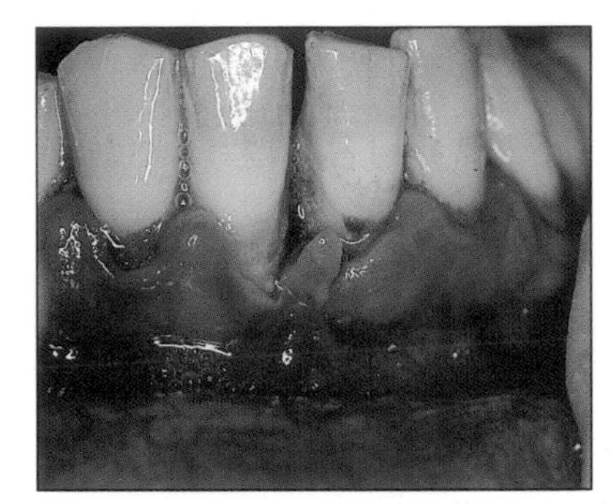

Appalling oral hygiene and periodontitis in a patient awaiting cardiac valvular surgery. Dental procedures involving gingival laceration or periodontal disruption (such as extraction) can produce bacteraemia of oral microorganisms, which could lead to infective endocarditis

Medically compromised patients

The commonest problems are in patients with a bleeding tendency or cardiovascular disease, or who are immunocompromised.

Bleeding disorders

Dental extractions and surgical procedures, including local analgesic injections, can cause problems in patients treated with anticoagulant drugs and those with coagulation defects or severe thrombocytopenic states.

With patients treated with anticoagulant drugs, local analgesia and minor surgery (simple extractions of two or three teeth) may generally be carried out safely in general practice with no change in treatment if test results are within the normal therapeutic range (international normalised ratio <3). The same is true for patients with thrombocytopenia if the platelet count exceeds $50 \times 10^9/l$. Postoperatively, a 4.8% tranexamic acid mouthwash, 10 ml used four times daily for a week, may help.

In all but severe cases of haemophilia, non-surgical dental treatment can be carried out on haemophilic patients under antifibrinolytic cover (tranexamic acid), though care must be taken to maintain urinary flow to avoid urinary blood clot problems. Haematological advice must be sought before other procedures are undertaken. With mild haemophilia, minor oral surgery may be possible under desmopressin (DDAVP) cover. In other cases factor replacement is necessary.

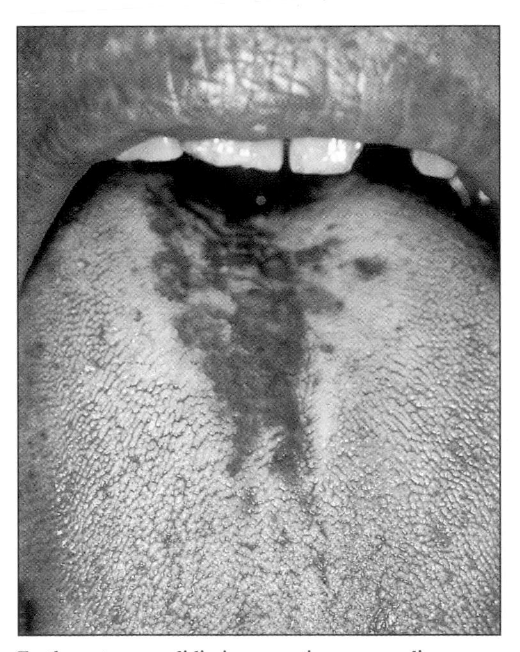

Erythematous candidiasis, presenting as a median rhomboid glossitis, is common in patients with immune defects

In patients with bleeding disorders

- **Surgery can be hazardous in bleeding states**
- **Haemophilic patients need factor replacement before most surgery**
- **Patients treated with anticoagulant drugs can usually safely undergo minor procedures if the international normalised ratio <3**
- **Thrombocytopenic patients can usually safely undergo minor procedures if platelet count is over $50 \times 10^9/l$**
- **Tranexamic mouthwashes used postoperatively may help haemostasis**
- **Good oral care and hygiene are essential**

Cardiovascular disease

Ischaemic heart disease

It is generally accepted that routine dentistry for most patients with ischaemic heart disease should be undertaken using short appointments and under local analgesia. More complex surgical procedures should be carried out in hospital with full cardiac monitoring. Elective dental care for patients who have recently had a myocardial infarct should be deferred for at least three months, and some recommend a delay of 12 months.

Cardiac pacemakers
The chief hazards from dental equipment to pacemakers are from electrosurgery and diathermy, but these are infrequently used and the risk from other equipment such as ultrasonic scalers or pulp testers is very small.

Cardiac valvular defects
Tooth extractions and dental procedures involving the periodontium can produce a bacteraemia of oral microorganisms, especially *Streptococcus mutans* and *S sanguis*, which can lead to infective endocarditis in patients at risk. However, dental treatment precedes only 10-15% of diagnosed cases, and in real terms the risks are thought to be fairly remote.

Oral health care (including maintaining high levels of oral hygiene) should be completed before valvular surgery. It is considered prudent to provide antibiotic cover for patients at risk who are about to have extractions, periodontal surgery, mucogingival flaps raised (oral surgery), scaling, tooth reimplantation, or other procedures where there is gingival laceration. However, there is no convincing evidence for the need for antibiotic prophylaxis for most local analgesic injections or for non-surgical, prosthetic, restorative, or orthodontic procedures other than banding or debanding.

The current basic recommendations are to use a chlorhexidine mouthwash and, one hour before the dental procedure, a single oral dose of 3 g of amoxicillin (or 600 mg clindamycin for patients allergic to penicillin). Patients with a history of infective endocarditis require intravenous antibiotic prophylaxis.

In patients with cardiac valvular defects
- **Good oral care and hygiene are essential**
- **Oral healthcare screening and treatment should be completed before valvular surgery**
- **Antimicrobial prophylaxis is indicated before invasive dental procedures**

Immunocompromised patients

Oral diseases in immunocompromised people tend to be more common with poor oral hygiene, malnutrition, and tobacco use. The commonest lesions are candidiasis and herpes viral infections, but others include ulcers, periodontal disease, and malignant neoplasms. Purpura and spontaneous gingival bleeding also are seen in patients with leukaemia. Drugs such as ciclosporin can cause gingival swelling.

Oral lesions in patients with HIV infection or AIDS are most likely to appear when the CD4 cell count is low and are often controlled, at least temporarily, by antiretroviral treatment. Anti-HIV drugs can cause oral problems such as ulcers, xerostomia, and salivary gland swelling. Oral features are now classified as strongly, less commonly, or possibly associated with HIV infection.

WHO classification of oral lesions in HIV infection and AIDS

Group I. Lesions strongly associated with HIV infection
- Candidiasis
  Erythematous
  Hyperplastic
  Thrush (pseudomembranous)
- Hairy leucoplakia (Epstein-Barr virus)
- HIV-gingivitis
- Necrotising ulcerative gingivitis
- HIV-periodontitis.
- Kaposi's sarcoma
- Non-Hodgkin's lymphoma

Group II. Lesions less commonly associated with HIV infection
- Atypical ulceration (oropharyngeal)
- Idiopathic thrombocytopenic purpura
- Salivary gland diseases
- Dry mouth
  Unilateral or bilateral swelling of major salivary glands
- Viral infections (except Epstein-Barr virus)
  Cytomegalovirus
  Herpes simplex virus
  Human papillomavirus (wart-like lesions)—condyloma acuminatum, focal epithelial hyperplasia, verruca vulgaris
- Varicella-zoster virus—herpes zoster and varicella

Group III. Lesions possibly associated with HIV infection.
- Miscellany of rare diseases

Candidiasis
Thrush and erythematous candidiasis are common in patients with immune defects and are often an early manifestation of the immunodeficiency. There is an increase, especially in those with HIV infection or AIDS, in antifungal resistance of *Candida albicans* and in non-albicans species such as *C krusei* and new species such as *C dubliniensis* and *C inconspicua*. Fluconazole in high doses, however, is often still effective.

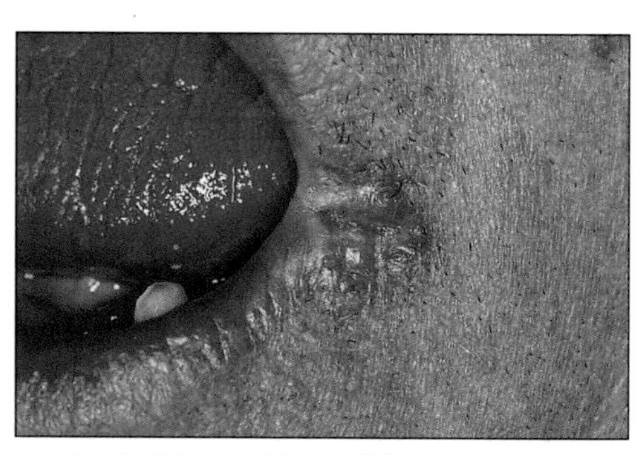

Angular cheilitis caused by candidiasis

Viral infections
Herpesviruses, especially herpes simplex virus, may cause herpes labialis, or oral or perioral ulcers. Hairy leucoplakia, a common corrugated (or "hairy") white lesion, is usually seen in HIV infection or AIDS but may be seen in any immunocompromising state.

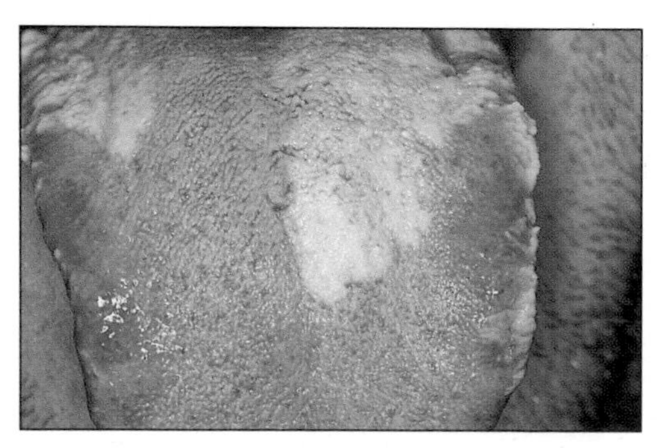

Hairy leucoplakia may be seen in immunocompromised patients

Mouth ulcers
Ulcers in immunocompromised persons may be related to aphthous type ulcers, infections (herpesviruses, mycoses (especially histoplasmosis or cryptococcosis), mycobacteria or

syphilis, or protozoa such as leishmaniasis), malignant neoplasms (see below), or drugs (such as cytotoxic or antiretroviral agents).

Diagnosis can be difficult, and biopsy with microbial studies may be needed to exclude infections such as cytomegalovirus or deep mycoses. Specific treatments are often indicated. Chlorhexidine and topical analgesics can be helpful local treatments. Granulocyte colony stimulating factor or thalidomide can be helpful in HIV related aphthous-like ulceration.

In immunocompromised patients
- **Oral candidiasis is common, and antifungal drugs are indicated**
- **Oral hairy leucoplakia is common in patients with AIDS; Epstein-Barr virus is implicated, but treatment is rarely indicated**
- **Mouth ulcers are common, and a wide range of aetiologies is possible**
- **Kaposi's sarcoma, lymphomas, and carcinomas may be seen**

Gingival and periodontal disease
Necrotising ulcerative gingivitis and periodontitis occur disproportionately often in immunocompromised patients for the level of oral hygiene. They can be painful and cause rapid loss of alveolar bone. Improved oral hygiene, debridement, chlorhexidine, and sometimes metronidazole are needed.

Malignant neoplasms
Immunocompromising conditions predispose patients to oral leucoplakia and carcinoma (see earlier articles), Kaposi's sarcoma, and lymphomas.

Kaposi's sarcoma typically occurs on the palate or maxillary gingivae and presents as red, blue, or purple macules that progress to papules, nodules, or ulcers. It is associated with human herpesvirus 8. It can respond badly to irradiation but responds transiently to chemotherapy. Oral lesions are often managed with intralesional vinblastine or systemic chemotherapy if there are extraoral lesions.

Lymphomas are typically non-Hodgkin's lymphomas in the maxillary gingivae or fauces. They are part of widespread disease and are usually associated with Epstein-Barr virus. They are resistant to treatment, and chemotherapy is required.

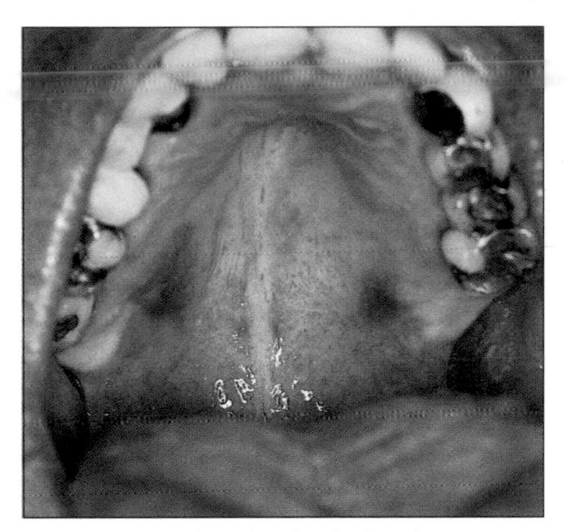

Kaposi's sarcomas in typical sites in the palate

Immunosuppressed patients and those with indwelling peritoneal catheters
Dental procedures are rarely followed by infection of such patients, and any infections rarely involve oral microorganisms. Thus, patients do not require antimicrobial prophylaxis before routine dental procedures unless they have a severe immune defect, there is some other indication, or surgery is to be performed.

Patients with artificial joints
Joint prostheses are only rarely infected because of dental procedures or oral microorganisms. Thus, patients with artificial joints do not require antimicrobial prophylaxis before most dental procedures unless there is some other indication, although antimicrobial use may be prudent for the first two years after arthroplasty and in patients with inflammatory arthropathies or who are immunocompromised.

In immunocompromised patients or those with prosthetic joints
- **Good oral care and hygiene are essential**
- **Antimicrobial prophylaxis is not usually necessary before dental procedures**

Mentally challenged patients

Mentally challenged people often have poor oral health (missing or discoloured teeth, periodontal disease, and oral malodour), which worsens their struggle for social acceptance. Barriers to dental treatment include fear (aggravated by inability to comprehend the need for treatment), the need to be accompanied, difficult access to healthcare facilities, and often a negative attitude or lack of training of the professional.

Patients with a mild to moderate disability can often be treated in general dental practice with help and encouragement from relatives and carers. Recent guidelines issued by the General Dental Council on minimum standards for general

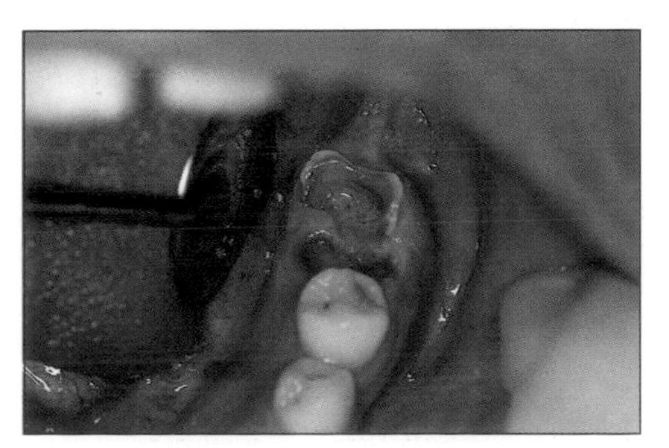

Poor oral condition in a mentally challenged person

anaesthesia will probably lead to a decline in the availability of this in general practice. Those who require additional resources are often treated in the community dental service. For the most severely affected patients, dental care may have to be performed under general anaesthesia or intravenous sedation, often only available in the community dental service or hospital.

In mentally challenged patients
- **Good oral care and hygiene are essental**
- **Access to care is often limited**
- **Preoperative sedation may be needed**

Patients with mental illness

People with mental illness often avoid dental care, and their oral hygiene may be impaired, with consequential periodontal disease and caries. Their medication may produce adverse oral effects, especially xerostomia (with increased risk of caries) and dyskinesias. Dental management commonly involves ensuring good oral health care (which may involve the support of a carer), delaying treatment until there is relative psychiatric equilibrium, keeping appointments short, and oral or intravenous sedation as required.

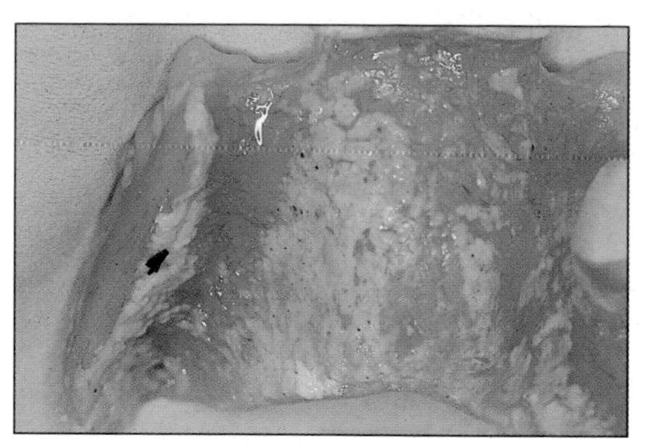

Uncleaned denture in a person with psychiatric illness

Socially excluded patients

Overall, oral health in UK children has been improving, and these benefits should soon be reflected among adults. However, the inequalities in oral health and in the use of services have increased between affluent and deprived groups, especially socially excluded groups (institutionalised elderly people, homeless people, refugees and asylum seekers, those engaged in substance misuse, etc).

Institutionalised elderly people are more likely to have fewer teeth but more gross caries and root caries than other elderly groups.

Homeless people often are not registered for dental care, make little use of dental services, miss dental appointments, have poor oral health, and are at increased risk of oral cancer.

Refugees and asylum seekers often find access to dental services difficult.

People who engage in substance misuse often have poor oral hygiene; tend to prefer sweet foods and sugar (especially methadone users), leading to caries; have damaged or lost teeth because of convulsions; and make little use of dental services, about which they have high anxiety.

In socially excluded people
- **Oral health is often poor**
- **Access to oral health care is impeded**
- **Good oral care and hygiene are essential**

Further reading

- Aartman IH, de Jongh A, Makkes PC, Hoogstraten J. Treatment modalities in a dental fear clinic and the relation with general psychopathology and oral health variables. *Br Dent J* 1999;186: 467-71
- Academy of Dentistry for Persons with Disabilities. A position paper from the Academy of Dentistry for Persons with Disabilities: preservation of quality oral health care services for people with developmental disabilities. *Spec Care Dentist* 1998;18:180-2
- Bedi R, Uppal RDK. The oral health of minority ethnic communities in the United Kingdom. *Br Dent J* 1995;179:421-5
- Carter EF. Dental implications of narcotic addiction. *Aust Dent J* 1978;23:308-10
- Hakeberg M, Dernevik L, Gatzinsky P, Eklof C, Kennergren C, Jontell M. The significance of oral health and dental treatment for the postoperative outcome of heart valve surgery. *Scand Cardiovasc J* 1999;33:5-8
- Porter SR, Scully C, eds. *Oral healthcare for those with HIV and other special needs.* Northwood: Science Reviews, 1995.
- Scully C, Flint S, Porter SR. *Oral diseases.* London: Martin Dunitz, 1996
- Yilmaz S, Ozlu Y, Ekuklu G. The effect of dental training on the reactions of mentally handicapped children's behavior in the dental office. *ASDC J Dent Child* 1999;66:154-5, 188-9

10 Dental emergencies

Graham Roberts, Crispian Scully, Rosemary Shotts

Most oral emergencies relate to pain, bleeding, or orofacial trauma and should be attended by a dental practitioner. However, in the absence of access to dental care, a medical practitioner may be called on to help. Jaw fractures require the attention of oral or maxillofacial surgeons.

Dental pain

Pulpal pain is spontaneous, strong, often throbbing, and exacerbated by temperature and outlasts the evoking stimulus. Localisation is poor, and pain tends to radiate to the ipsilateral ear, temple, or cheek. The pain may abate spontaneously, but the patient should still be referred for dental advice, as the pulp has probably necrosed, and acute periapical periodontitis (dental abscess) will probably follow in due course. Endodontics (root canal treatment) or tooth extraction are required.

Periapical periodontitis pain is spontaneous and severe, persists for hours, is well localised, and is exacerbated by biting. The adjacent gum is often tender to palpation. An abscess may form ("gumboil"), sometimes with facial swelling, fever, and illness. Fascial space infections are fortunately rare since they threaten the airway: patients should be referred to a specialist. In the absence of immediate dental attention it is best to incise a fluctuant abscess and give antimicrobials (amoxicillin) and analgesics. The acute situation usually then resolves, but the abscess will recur, since the necrotic pulp will become re-infected unless the tooth is endodontically treated or extracted, though a chronic abscess may be asymptomatic apart from a discharging sinus. Rarely, this may open on to the skin.

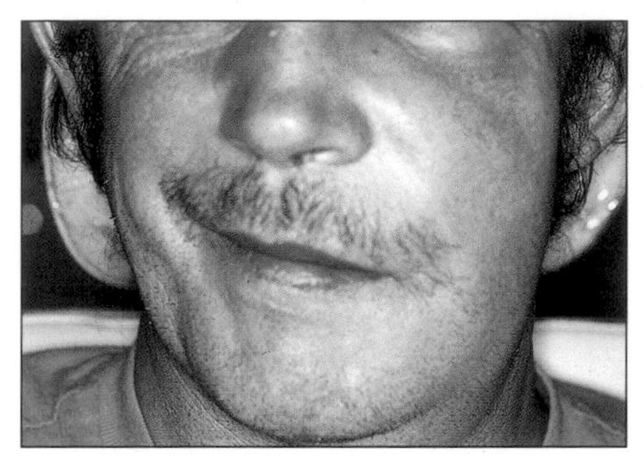

Orofacial swelling in a patient with an acute dental abscess

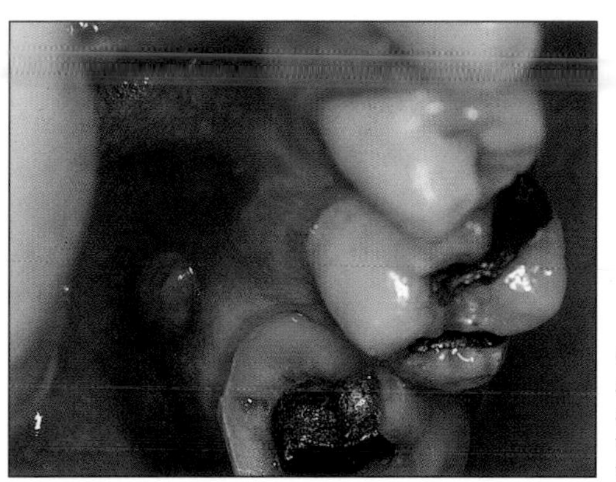

Chronic dental abscess (gumboil) at a typical site, in this case related to the broken molar

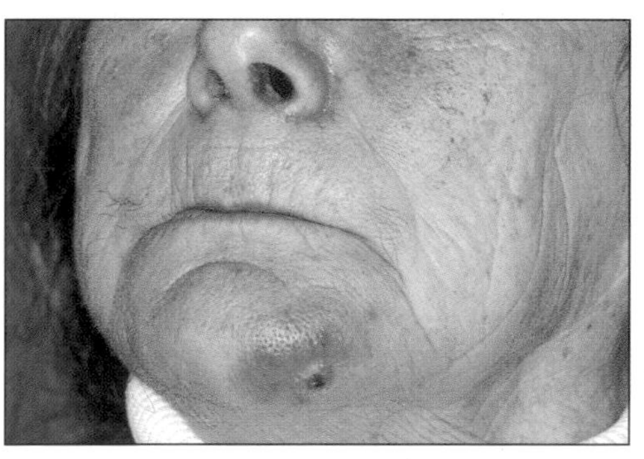

Dental sinus opening on to skin

- **Emergency treatment of dental abscess is antimicrobials, analgesics, and drainage of a fluctuant swelling by a dentist**
- **Dental treatment should then be arranged, or the abscess will recur**

Bleeding

Most oral bleeding results from gingivitis (see earlier article) or trauma, but if it is prolonged consider a bleeding tendency.

Trauma

After a tooth is extracted, the socket bleeds normally for a few minutes but then clots. Since clots are easily disturbed, patients should be advised not to rinse their mouth, disturb the clot, chew hard, take hot drinks or alcohol, or exercise for the next 24 hours. If the socket continues to bleed lie a gauze pad across the socket and ask the patient to bite on it for 15-30 minutes. If it is still bleeding place Surgicel or another haemostatic agent in the socket. If the bleeding continues suture the socket and, lastly, consider a bleeding tendency.

- **Emergency care of post-extraction bleeding is to have the patient bite on gauze for 15-30 minutes**
- **Persistent bleeding may require packing the socket with a haemostatic agent or suturing, but it occasionally signifies an unrecognised bleeding tendency**

Dental indications for urgent admission to hospital

Trauma
- Middle facial third fractures
- Mandibular fractures unless simple or undisplaced
- Zygomatic fractures where there is danger of ocular damage

Inflammatory lesions and infections
- Cervical or facial fascial space infection
- Oral infections where patient is "toxic" or severely immunocompromised
- Tuberculosis (some)
- Severe viral infections
- Severe vesiculobullous disorders (pemphigus, Stevens-Johnson syndrome, toxic epidermal necrolysis)

Blood loss
- Severe or persistent haemorrhage (particularly in patient with a bleeding tendency)

Others
- Diabetes with poor control

Surgical complications

Post-extraction pain
Some pain and swelling after tooth extraction are common but ease over a few hours. Paracetamol usually provides adequate analgesia. Pain from complex procedures may last longer and should be controlled with regularly administered analgesics. If pain persists or increases the patient should return to the dentist to exclude pathology (such as dry socket or jaw fracture).

Infection
Localised osteitis (dry socket) occasionally follows an extraction, typically a lower molar extraction. After two to four days there is usually increasing pain, halitosis, unpleasant taste, an empty socket, and tenderness. Exclude retained roots, foreign body, jaw fracture, osteomyelitis, or other pathology, especially if there is fever, intense pain, or neurological signs such as labial anaesthesia. Treat by irrigating with warm (50°C) saline or aqueous chlorhexidine, dressing the socket (several concoctions are available), and giving analgesics and antimicrobials (metronidazole).

Actinomycosis a rare late complication of extraction or jaw fracture and usually presents as a chronic purplish swelling. A three week course of penicillin is often indicated.

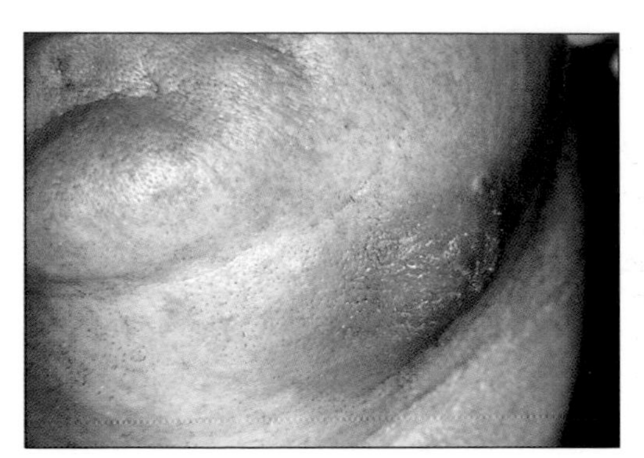

Actinomycosis

- **Pain increasing after an extraction may indicate infection or fracture**
- **Radiograph to exclude pathology**
- **Irrigate and dress the socket, and consider antimicrobials and analgesics**

Antral complications
Loss of tooth or root into the antrum—Give antimicrobials and a nasal decongestant and locate the object by radiography. A further operation is required.

Oroantral fistula—Patients should not blow their nose. Antimicrobials and nasal decongestants help. If it is detected early, primary closure is possible, but others may need flap closure by a specialist.

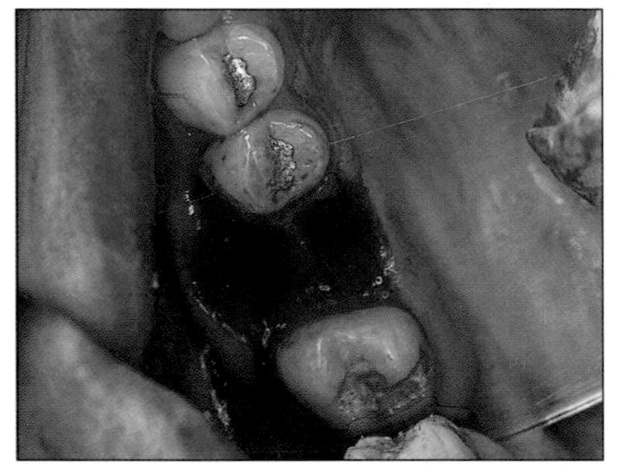

Oroantral fistula after extraction of an upper molar. The antral floor is often in close proximity to the roots of maxillary molars and premolars

Fractured teeth

Injuries to the primary teeth may be of little consequence with regard to emergency care, but even seemingly mild injuries can damage the permanent successors. Upwards of 30% of children damage their permanent teeth by the age of 15.

Enamel fracture needs no emergency care, but dental attention should be sought later. More severe injuries affecting the dentine should be treated as urgent as there might be pulpal infection. Emergency care consists of placing a suitable dentine lining material on to the fractured dentine, and so prompt treatment by a dentist within the same working day or at least by the following morning is required. Fractured roots require dental advice.

Avulsed teeth

Avulsed permanent anterior teeth can be replanted successfully in a child, particularly if the root apex is not completely formed (under 16 years old). Avulsed primary teeth should not be replanted. The younger the child and the sooner the replantation, the better the success; teeth replanted within 15 minutes stand a 98% chance of being retained after further dental attention.

Immediate replantation gives the best results. Hold the tooth by the crown (do not handle root as that could damage the periodontal ligament). If the tooth is contaminated rinse it with sterile saline, and if the socket contains a clot remove it with saline irrigation. Replant the tooth the right way round (ensure the labial (convex) surface is facing forward) and manually compress the socket. Splint the tooth; "finger crimping" a foil milk bottle top is a temporary measure, an alternative is tissue adhesive. The child should see a dentist within 72 hours.

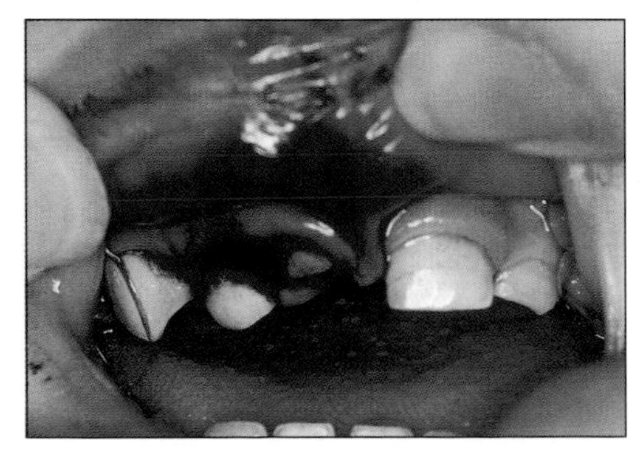

Oral and dental trauma after a skateboarding accident

If immediate replantation is not possible place tooth in an isotonic fluid (cool fresh pasteurised or long life milk, saline, or contact lens fluid). Otherwise, if the child is cooperative, place tooth in the buccal sulcus and get to a dentist within 30 minutes. Unsuitable and slightly damaging fluids are water (because of isotonic damage as a result of prolonged exposure), disinfectants, bleach, and fruit juice. The use of a doxycycline immersion before reimplantation by the dentist may be helpful in preventing later external root resorption.

Splint the tooth for 7-10 days, with no biting on splinted teeth, soft diet, and good oral hygiene.

Follow up—Root resorption, ankylosis, and tooth submergence (infraocclusion) are potential complications.

- **Primary teeth should not be replanted**
- **Permanent teeth in children can be successfully replanted**
- **Hold tooth by crown, keep clean and moist in saline or milk, replant as soon as possible, and splint**

Maxillofacial trauma

Dislocation or subluxation of mandible

This is commonly caused by a blow to the chin when the jaw is open. The condyles are dislocated forwards and upwards anterior to the eminence, and the patient gags open.

Fractures must be excluded. Reduction can usually be achieved by facing the patient and placing the thumb pads over the lower molars and applying downwards pressure and simultaneously, with the fingers under the chin, rotating the jaw backwards and upwards. If muscle spasm prevents reduction intravenous midazolam may be needed. After reduction, wide opening of the jaw should be avoided.

Recurrent dislocation is a feature of Ehlers-Danlos and Marfan's syndromes.

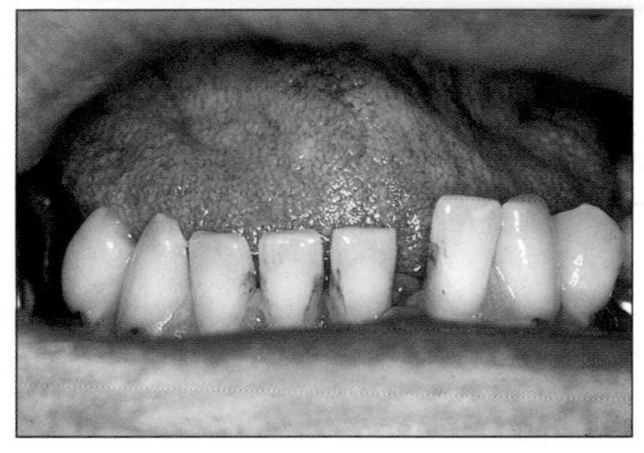

Step deformity of occlusion revealing mandibular fracture

Jaw fractures

These mainly result from high velocity impact as in road traffic accidents, other accidents, and assaults.

The immediate concern is to preserve the airway. Assess all traumatised patients along the lines of the advanced trauma life support scheme (ATLS). Other immediate life threatening problems include intracranial haemorrhage, severe haemorrhage from other sites, and cervical spine damage. During the secondary survey, inspect the head for lacerations and leakage of cerebrospinal fluid.

Associated bleeding may further compromise the airway. Jaw fractures alone, unless associated with a split palate or gunshot wounds, rarely cause severe haemorrhage. Bleeding from a ruptured inferior dental artery usually stops spontaneously, but may recur if, for example, there is traction on the mandible. Severe maxillofacial bleeding may be tamponaded with craniofacial fixation. Bleeding can arise from fractured nasal bones, in which case nasal packing may be required. If bleeding recurs the damaged vessel must be ligated.

Definitive management of fractures, despite frighteningly severe disfigurement, is not an immediate priority, but debris such as fractured teeth, blood, and saliva should be cleared from the mouth, and the tongue may be controlled by a dorsal suture. An oropharyngeal airway may be required. Involve the maxillofacial team early on for treatment planning.

Intubation may be necessary in presence of substantial head injury, and inability to intubate may necessitate surgical cricothyroidotomy, since nasotracheal intubation is contraindicated.

The diagnosis of fracture is from the history, pain, swelling, bruising (haematoma), bleeding (usually intraorally), mobility of fragments (and crepitus), deranged occlusion, paraesthesia or anaesthesia of nerves involved, and radiographic signs.

Radiographs for demonstrating maxillofacial fractures

Mandibular fracture
- Panoramic *or*
- Bilateral oblique laterals
- Postero-anterior view of mandible
- Occlusal

Temporomandibular joint and condyle fracture
- Conventional and high orthopantomogram *or*
- Reverse Towne's
- Consider computed tomography

Zygomatic arch fracture
- Occipitomental
- Submentovertex (exposed for zygomatic arches, not base of skull)

Middle third fracture
- Occipitomental 30°
- Occipitomental 10°
- Lateral skull
- Computed tomography

Skull fracture
- Postero-anterior view of skull
- Lateral skull (brow up)
- Submentovertex (exposed for base of skull)
- Computed tomography

Nasal fracture
- Soft tissues lateral view for nasal bones
- Occipitomental 30°

Mandibular fractures

These are commonly owing to assault and are usually simple and not associated with serious other injuries or bleeding. If the symphysis is comminuted the tongue could fall back and obstruct the airway, and this must be prevented. Simple undisplaced fractures may occasionally be treated conservatively with a soft diet if the teeth are not damaged. If the fragments are excessively mobile, pain will be substantial, and early fixation is the best management. Most fractures are managed by open reduction and internal fixation, usually with mini-plates.

Middle third or upper facial skeleton fractures

These commonly arise from severe trauma (particularly road traffic accidents) and are classified into Le Fort fracture lines:
I—Low level above the nasal floor (swelling of upper lip)
II—Subzygomatic (massive swelling of face: ballooning) (Panda facies)
III—Suprazygomatic (massive swelling of face and cerebrospinal rhinorrhoea).

There may be airway obstruction, head injury, chest injuries, ruptured viscera, and fractured spine and long bones. Most middle third fractures are treated by open reduction and internal fixation with mini-plates.

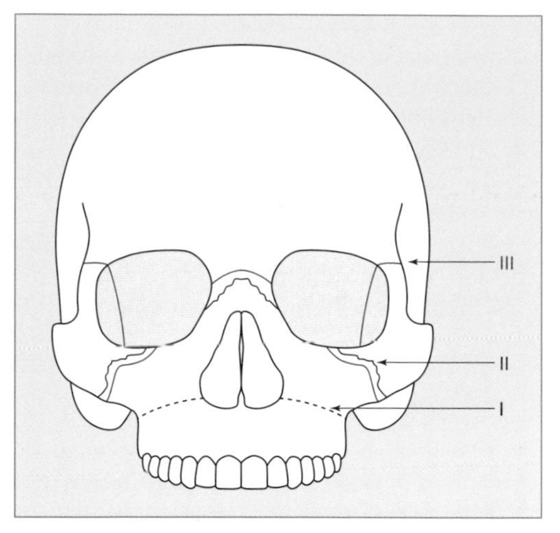

Le Fort lines of middle third facial fractures (redrawn from Scully et al. *Oxford Handbook of Dental Patient Care.* Oxford University Press, 1998)

Zygomatic (malar) fractures

These are typically due to assaults. Orbital features are common and include depression of cheek, lateral subconjunctival haemorrhage, rim step deformities, restricted eye movements, changes in visual acuity, variation in pupil size and reactivity, and, occasionally, enophthalmos or exophthalmos.

Undisplaced uncomplicated fractures need no treatment but should be reviewed as early as possible within two weeks. For others, reduction is by elevating from the temporal region (Gillies approach), an intraoral approach, or open reduction and internal fixation.

- **The priority in patients with maxillofacial injury is the airway**
- **Middle third facial fractures may be associated with cerebrospinal rhinorrhoea**
- **Zygomatic fractures may be associated with ocular damage**
- **The maxillofacial team should be involved at an early stage for planning treatment**

Further reading

- Andreasen JO, Andreasen FM. *Textbook and colour atlas of traumatic injuries to the teeth.* Copenhagen: Munksgaard, 1994
- Bishop BG, Donnelly JC. Proposed criteria for classifying potential dental emergencies in Department of Defence military personnel. *Mil Med* 1997;162:130-5
- Gilthorpe MS, Wilson RC, Moles DR, Bedi R. Variations in admissions to hospital for head injury and assault to the head. Part 1: Age and gender. *Br J Oral Maxillofac Surg* 1999;37:294-300
- Moles DR, Gilthorpe MS, Wilson RC, Bedi R. Variations in admission to hospital for head injury and assault to the head. Part 2: Ethnic group. *Br J Oral Maxillofac Surg* 1999;37:301-8
- Muthukrishnan A, Walters H, Douglas PS. An audit of antibiotic prescribing by general practitioners in the initial management of acute dental infection. *Dent Update* 1996;23:316-8
- Nelson LP, Shusterman S. Emergency management of oral trauma in children. *Curr Opin Pediatr* 1997;9:242-5
- Roberts G, Longhurst P. *Oral and dental trauma in children and adolescents.* Oxford: Oxford University Press, 1996
- Sheller B, Williams BJ, Lombardi SM. Diagnosis and treatment of dental caries-related emergencies in a children's hospital. *Pediatr Dent* 1997;19:470-5

Index

Page numbers in **bold** refer to figures; those in *italic* to tables or boxed material